TRANSPERSONAL MEDICINE

TRANSPERSONAL MEDICINE

The New Approach to Healing
Body-Mind-Spirit

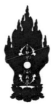

G. Frank Lawlis, PH.D.

FOREWORD BY
Larry Dossey, M.D.

SHAMBHALA
Boston & London
1996

Shambhala Publications, Inc.
Horticultural Hall
300 Massachusetts Avenue
Boston, Massachusetts 02115

Chapter 11 is an excerpt from an early draft of
Dancing with Cancer (Dallas: Noteman Press, 1995),
© 1994, 1995 by Robert Elliott. Used with the author's permission.

9 8 7 6 5 4 3 2 1

First Edition
Printed in the United States of America
⊗ This edition is printed on acid-free paper that meets the
American National Standards Institute Z39.48 Standard.

ISBN 1-57062-626-X

Library of Congress Cataloging-in-Publication Data
Lawlis, G. Frank.
Transpersonal medicine: the new approach to healing body-mind-
spirit / by G. Frank Lawlis; foreword by Larry Dossey. — 1st ed.
p. cm.

1. Mental healing. 2. Transpersonal psychology 3. Medicine and
psychology. 4. Mind and body. I. Title.
RZ401.L285 1996   95-48803
615.8'52—dc20   CIP

To Jeanne, the Goddess

CONTENTS

II. *Beyond the Self in Vertical Space*

III. *Special Issues*

> , , ,

FOREWORD

CONFIDENCE IS RUNNING HIGH in medicine these days. We hear that we're homing in on the ultimate determinants of disease, including the genes themselves. As we penetrate our DNA we will learn how to rearrange it, and soon all the maladies of humankind will be on the run. As a fan of scientific medicine, I applaud these developments. But an increasing number of people within the profession, myself included, believe that a continued physical approach to human health is unlikely to issue in utopia. The main reason is that something has been left out, something that counts as a first principle: mind or consciousness.

Dr. Frank Lawlis's book is about this missing factor. Lawlis has explored this area for three decades and is well qualified to speak about it. This in itself is nothing new; other veterans have also written books on the role of the mind in health. But Lawlis's book is different because of the multifaceted ways in which he approaches the mind. The result is an infinitely richer and scientifically more accurate picture of the role of consciousness in health.

Currently, most medical researchers insist that consciousness is only a byproduct of the chemistry, anatomy, and physiology of the brain (never mind how this happens; the experts don't know). As one authority in the field of artificial intelligence put it, the brain is simply a computer made of meat. This materialistic point of view has a deadening effect on the belief that there is anything "higher" than the physical brain and body. If the experts are right—if consciousness is all physical—the transpersonal, spiritual dimension is an illusion.

Why speak, then, of a transpersonal domain and of a transpersonal medicine that go "beyond the person"? The reason comes, surprisingly, from science itself. Today hundreds of scientific studies strongly suggest that, to put it simply, consciousness can do things that brains cannot do. This means that the mind must be, in some sense, more than the brain and body. Experiments suggest, for example, that consciousness can act *nonlocally*, at a distance, without mediation by any detectable form of energy. These studies show that the effects of consciousness do not get weaker with distance, and that they cannot be shielded or blocked by any known physical barrier. The evidence indicates that nonlocal mental influences are not "caused" in any conventional sense. Summing up this body of knowledge, physicist Nick Herbert, an expert in the field of nonlocality, attributes three distinguishing qualities to nonlocal events. They are *unmediated, unmitigated,* and *immediate.* As a result of these findings we are confronted with a radically new view of the mind—mind as *nonlocal*—mind not localized to points in space, such as brains or bodies, or to points in time, such as the present moment.

A key realization is that nonlocal does not mean "very large," "a long way off," or "a very long time." Nonlocality implies *infinitude* in space and time. Therefore, if some aspect of the mind is genuinely nonlocal, it is omnipresent and immortal—characteristics of what Westerners have loosely called the soul, perhaps what Buddhists call Buddha nature. Nonlocal qualities also imply an indwelling divine aspect of humans, because we have always associated omnipresence and immortality with the Absolute. The spiritual implications of the nonlocal view are profound and are explored by Frank Lawlis in this book.

Several categories of transpersonal mental phenomena have far-reaching implications for health and healing. These include transpersonal imagery, distant or intercessory prayer, intuitive or distant diagnosis, telesomatic events in which distant individuals share physical symptoms, and many other types of events explored in these pages. These examples may seem disparate and unrelated, but they have at least one feature in common: love. Empathy, compassion, and deep caring appear to catalyze distant, nonlocal events between human beings.

We need to be attentive to how the field of transpersonal medicine is languaged. We should be especially careful in how we communicate these concepts to colleagues and skeptics, who may not have a feel for them or who may actually be hostile. An important point to bear in mind is that *transpersonal* and *nonlocal* are not identical and interchangeable terms. Importantly, if an event can be explained in terms of everyday sensory stimuli—energetic exchanges in the see-touch-feel world—it is not a nonlocal occurrence. If a transpersonal event is described as nonlocal, it must behave like a nonlocal event. It must be unmediated by any known energetic signal, not subject to dissipation with increasing spatial separation, incapable of being shielded or blocked by physical barriers, and so on. Moreover, transpersonal events involve persons; nonlocal events can also occur between persons but between inanimate objects such as electrons and photons as well.

If this sounds like needless haggling over terms, one has only to look at certain disciplines within the field of alternative medicine to see why the vocabulary one chooses is critical. As two examples, the imprecise use of the term *energy* by practitioners of Therapeutic Touch has led to vicious criticism by skeptics. The use of *subluxation* in chiropractic has led to similar criticism. Postulating transpersonal phenomena will arouse enough ire; we do not need to add to it by slippages of language.

We should resist equating "transpersonal" and "nonlocal" with "spiritual." Although transpersonal and nonlocal experiences are often associated with the feeling that there is "something greater" and "something more," this is not always the case. There is nothing necessarily "spiritual" about any of these dimensions. Experiencing states of being that are beyond space and time may entail spiritual feelings but "also sounds like passing out," as transpersonal psychologist Ken Wilber wryly states. Sudden and unanticipated immersion in these experiences is not always pleasant and rewarding. Thus it is said, "The unwise drown in the sea in which the mystic swims." That is why personal psychological work should ideally precede or go hand in hand with transpersonal work.

The reward of transpersonal medicine is different from that of physically based, orthodox medicine, which focuses on elimination and sometimes the prevention of disease. The ultimate goal of transpersonal medicine is realizing one's inherent completeness and divinity. This understanding has been variously called enlightenment, *nirvana*, *moksha*, and so on. Transpersonal medicine is, then, an invitation to see ourselves in a radically new way, and to take literally the reminders from practically every major religion that we are indeed divine—for example, from Hinduism, *"Tat tvam asi!"* ("Thou art that!).

This brings us to the greatest paradox of transpersonal medicine. If, in some sense, we are immortal and divine, why be concerned with health and longevity? Why not? It is nowhere written that, when we contact our transpersonal, eternal, nonlocal self, we have to renounce our local identity—our bodies, our flesh—and our concern with physical health. The ancient Taoists, who were highly attuned to their immortal Self, were intensely interested in living long lives. The transpersonal vision can coexist with the local, limited ways of seeing ourselves. Likewise, transpersonal medicine can cohabit with orthodox therapies. We are not required, on contacting our higher self, to invade the hospitals, unhook all the IVs, and unplug the ventilators. But if we choose not to use these therapies, we do so not with a sense of fear and impending doom but with a sense of celebration—realizing that, when we die, our most essential Self survives. Therefore, transpersonal medicine is Eternity Medicine, a form of therapy that goes beyond temporality; and practitioners of transpersonal medicine are not internists, they are eternists.

One of Lawlis's many keen insights is his caution that spiritual wisdom and physical health do not always go hand in hand. One can be spiritually enlightened and get *very* sick. The Buddha—the Awakened One—died of food poisoning; Job, who was "perfect" (Job 1:1), was afflicted with a terrible disease. Sri Ramana Maharshi, the most beloved saint of modern India, died of stomach cancer; Jesus Christ died of acute trauma. To equate spiritual achievement with physical perfection is a great temptation, but there is no historic or clinical justification for this point of view. Transpersonal medicine may lead to a longer, healthier life, but it is fundamentally "trans" these concerns. So let us use transpersonal medicine to encourage the cancer to go away or the heart attack to heal. But if they do not, and we die, we shall have to settle for immortality—not a bad consolation prize.

Transpersonal medicine is a great Reclamation Act that restores meaning in health and illness. This is vitally important, for unless we make a place for meaning we cannot understand who lives and dies. Take, for instance, the death of Thomas Jefferson, the third president of the United States. Jefferson died on July 4th, the fiftieth anniversary of the signing of the Declaration of Independence, which he helped draft. His final words were, "Is it the Fourth?" John Adams, our second president, died on the same day. Skeptics might say, "Nothing special—both Jefferson and Adams had one in 365 chances of dying on July 4th." But surely their deaths *meant* something; they symbolized, represented, and stood for something transpersonal, something beyond the physical self. From Lawlis's perspective, perhaps all deaths are transpersonally significant. They point beyond the body; they reflect more than the blind play of atoms and molecules.

To get a glimpse of how far-reaching the transpersonal perspective can be, consider the commonest killer in our society, coronary artery disease. More individuals die from heart attacks on Monday morning, eight to nine AM, than at any other time of the week—the Black Monday syndrome. Surveys have shown that one of the best predictors of heart attacks in people under fifty is job dissatisfaction: the *meaning* of work, the *meaning* of a job. The fact that we die of heart disease more frequently on a particular day of the week is quite strange; as far as we know, human beings are the only species on earth that manages to do so. Humans, too, are the premier meaning-making species. Thus the need for "meaning therapies" such as those presented in this book, which can help us change negative meanings to positive ones.

This wise, insightful book is a valuable contribution. It is an indicator of the future of medicine. It shows that any medicine that does not honor and engage the transpersonal dimensions of human experience is limited and incomplete. As you read it, may you find greater meaning in your own life, and may you encounter your own divinity as well.

—*Larry Dossey*, M.D.

> , , ,

PREFACE

P RIOR TO HIS DEATH, Albert Einstein asked one of life's critical
questions: "Is the Universe kind?" An affirmative response to that
question implies that life events have meaning within the structural
context of a larger order. From this perspective, something that we
generally regard as "bad," such as disease, could be seen as a motivating force for change and transformation, and thus could be "kind."

How might such a philosophical question be applicable to a health
care industry that represents eleven percent of the gross national product and will grow to fifteen percent by the end of the century (with two
trillion dollars a year spent on health care)? If the answer to Einstein's
question is yes, then an individual's health care is a sacred and personal
growth experience. If all is random, then an illness is nothing more
than one of life's inconveniences, to be dealt with as impersonally and
quickly as possible. Currently, we live more often with the latter concept; our health care system reflects the random chaos of our perception of disease.

As we explore healing from a more historical, psychological, and
practical perspective than ever before, it becomes clear that humans,
as a species, did not suddenly develop the capacity to heal with the

advent of chemical technology. In fact, many scholars, such as Leonard Sagan in his book, *Health of Nations,* cast doubt on whether modern medicine has had any major effect on disease at all.[1] Perhaps we should study the older forms of healing as an avenue toward understanding this phenomenon. The immediate result of looking at ancient ways is the recognition of the role of consciousness as critical to all concepts of rejuvenation.

Yet many of the disciplines that study consciousness, such as psychology, have confined the role of mind to mechanistic phenomena as much as the physical sciences have. The first force in psychological philosophy, the behaviorists, posited that the basic motivation of humankind is to find the behavior that will most result in gratification. Like the rat learning the right response in order to get a food pellet, the individual perpetually looks for the right switch to bring about happiness. As the expectations change from one situation to another, the responses also change, so that the human challenge is to learn the systems quickly and efficiently in order to obtain total satisfaction.

The second force of psychology, the foundation of which is psychoanalysis, maintained that the crucial motivation of humankind is to resolve conflicting primal urges, societal structures, and personal satisfaction. Since these conflicts often arise in very early stages of life, much of later life is dedicated toward resolving the complexes that weave themselves around these issues.

The third force of psychological thought is humanistic psychology, with such proponents as Carl Rogers and Fritz Perls. This school holds the basic tenet that the motivational thrust of human development is the impetus to reach one's greatest "human potential." As one matures, one continually seeks out new nuances of self-discovery.

All three of these forces portray the developmental evolution of consciousness as circumscribed within the structure of the self and its relative energetic balance. The fourth force, transpersonal psychology, depicts evolutionary growth as coming from *beyond the self,* as a power larger or bigger than the individual, which implies a greater task to be accomplished, perhaps even at the expense of the self. The basic tenet of this approach is that the destiny of humanity is the evolution of the human spirit. As present needs are met, new ones emerge that challenge our hedonistic levels of satisfaction and move us toward those of higher spiritual value.

Transpersonal approaches assume within each individual planes of wisdom beyond the primary intellectual strength of the ego. They use therapeutic strategies that attempt to bring out from inner sources the knowledge of the unconscious. Transpersonal psychology tries to engage many levels of the personality for their valuable skills in dealing with particular issues. It views healing as the result of harmonizing and balancing the body-mind-spirit dynamics within a person's sphere of being. It holds that individual growth can be actualized through awareness and the utilization of mythic and symbolic imagery, incorporating cultural and personal dynamics.

The transpersonal approach also goes beyond the personal realm in enlisting support from others, considering the power of love and energetic resonance as important catalysts for change. It sees fellowship with others—community—as one of the strongest influences on our own transformational potential.

The following figure encapsulates the transpersonal orientation.

Inner World	*Outer World*
1. Boundaries of Self beyond time/space	1. Interpersonal boundaries beyond time/space
2. Evolving multiplicity of self into harmony	2. Evolving collective consciousness into awareness of interconnectedness
3. Mythical symbols link mind-body-spirit	3. Mythical symbols and intention of the collective empowers transformation

This book chronicles the pioneering efforts to apply this transpersonal orientation to the field of medicine. At its root, transpersonal medicine recognizes that the power of love, compassion, community, and intention are as important to healing as any of our pills and medicines, and possibly more powerful. If the health care system continues to stumble blindly without the awareness of the power of human consciousness, we will see the collapse of the faith of the people in the present institutions and watch them turn to those who offer something more than a seven-minute consultation and prescription. As systems of health care evolve, we will hopefully begin to appreciate the impact of transpersonal medicine from a cost-benefit and a quality-of-care basis.

As therapists and health care workers are called upon to find ways of promoting alternative levels of consciousness beyond the one of self-limitation, methodology based upon transpersonal philosophy has to be articulated, which is the aim of this book. Like a shaman's apprentice, one learns from masters and experienced teachers. With knowledge of the terrain of alternate worlds, a guide can better prepare and accompany the patient on his or her journey. The tools of the individual guide in the transpersonal realm include his or her knowledge of shifting states of consciousness, the therapeutic skills of counseling and caring, the abilities to genuinely express and receive love, and to orchestrate the power influence of a community. The shaman-therapist is also a storyteller and magician capable of weaving and changing the perceptions of reality for the person caught in cognitive traps.

The emerging awareness in all spheres of human life—medicine, business, family—is that the human experience includes many different levels of reality. An important component of the transpersonal approach is belief in the mystical relationship between humanity and the cosmos. In research and clinical findings, medical pioneers are defining methods and parameters for unique approaches that integrate this belief into treatment protocols and therapies. I hope that this book will serve as a guide for a new field of therapists, offering discussion and grounding for the validities of these approaches, as well as recognition of the mystery of the human soul.

ABOUT THIS BOOK

This book reviews the underlying principles of transpersonal medicine, with an emphasis on the treatment approaches that I have personally observed as effective for those wonderful patients with whom I have worked.

Part I focuses on ritual as a means of cross-personal empowerment.

After the introductory chapter, I describe important and powerful elements to be used in ritual building, including the practical technologies of creating sacred space. The third and fourth chapters provide descriptions of the nature of transpersonal imagery and the power that one person or group has upon the well-being of another when focusing on the other with love and compassion. These chapters contain the most direct manifestation of what we call the power of love, especially in terms of ritualizing change in positive ways.

Part II is devoted to the personal ritual, the process of empowering one's inner strengths and wisdoms. The first chapter within this section explores the ancient and modern skill of altering one's states of consciousness. This opening of the consciousness is the doorway to the wisdom beyond our usual state of mind. The second chapter within this section discusses personal ritual, which uses imagery as a language to understand the symbols and dynamics of the unconscious. Since we recognize the possibilities of multiple selves within one person, we also discuss the idea of the individual as a collective, a community within oneself.

Part III is dedicated to direct experiences and issues involved in medicine. There are three situations that are essentially transpersonal in nature and are common to all of us: the challenge of death, the transformative quality of humor, and the irritation and frustration of pain. These three aspects of human experience will be discussed in light of various transpersonal approaches. Finally, I present a case history that illustrates how these generalized issues led to the transformation of one human life.

Following each chapter is an interview with a leading researcher in the field of the topic discussed. These interviews allow the reader insight into the experiences of health care professionals applying transpersonal medicine approaches in a variety of ways.

I hope that this book will enrich the reader's quality of life—both physically and mentally—and bring to painful human ordeals the possibility of greater joy and peace. The book is grounded in the acknowledgment that health care is in crisis, and from purely a healing perspective, transpersonal medicine can be helpful because it offers practices that have significant applications to the survival of the individual who is in pain and suffering. Throughout the book, specific such applications are given.

Acknowledgments

This book has many midwives whom I would like to acknowledge. Most important to me and to the field is Jeanne Achterberg, my wife and colleague, who agented the work. I would also like to express my sincere appreciation and fondest thoughts to Emily Hilburn Sell, my editor and new-found West Texas ally, for her very hard work and patience in getting the manuscript into form. Of particular importance are my friends and colleagues—a *Who's Who* in the field, who contributed their comments and support to the project: Hal Bennett, Angeles Arrien, Charles Tart, Larry Dossey, Barbara Dossey, James Fadiman, Michael Harner, Stanley Krippner, Lawrence LeShan, Rachel Naomi Remen, Michael Samuels, Arthur Hastings, Robert Frager, Miles Vich, Dean Ornish, Carl Simonton, John Schneider, Robert Elliott, Jim McQuade, and Grandfather Raven. I also want to thank the wonderful friends and people I love who have healed me time and time again, and the wise patients who continue to teach me what life is all about.

⫶⫶ I ⫶⫶

BEYOND
THE SELF IN
HORIZONTAL
SPACE

⫼ 1 ⫼

TRANSPERSONAL
MEDICINE

*A New Paradigm in Understanding
the Healing of the Human Spirit*

ANYONE WHO HAS EVER spent much time in a hospital becomes acutely aware that life is a cycle of beginnings and endings, of birth and death, and sometimes rebirth. Although that realization is basic in our everyday lives as well, it is in medicine that it strikes us most dramatically. Nearly every day each one of us must confront endings and beginnings, large or small. It may be the end of a job or a relationship. It may be the death of a pet, a distant friend, or a significant loved one. There may be a birth in the family, an exciting new relationship, or a move to a new town.

As a psychologist working with people facing life-threatening illness or a future of physical impairment, I have become aware that facing such conditions with traditional psychological methods is not enough. I have been taught, for example, to help people *adjust* to life changes. But in most cases, adjustment means nothing more than changing roles, which all too often feels like, and is, a compromise for the patients; they sense, and I think rightly, that they are being asked to resign themselves to a lesser way of life.

3

What I have begun to see is that certain rare patients are able to do something much more than just "make an adjustment." Physical impairment, such as the loss of sight or a limb, allows them to abandon old ways of measuring self-worth and to set out on new journeys of self-discovery. In the process, they might assume social or career roles that to an outsider seem a step down, but that is not what has made their lives better. Their lives have improved because they have gotten in touch with a part of themselves that is much bigger than mere roles and much more important to them than their physical being. They have gotten in touch with new ways of valuing themselves and feeling valued, and these discoveries have radically changed the ways in which they relate to the world. They have begun relating not only through their bodies, or through the skills that once won them a certain role in life, but through their spiritual selves. Out of this awakening of their spiritual selves, they have begun to relate to the world in more loving ways, seeking, believing in, and connecting with other people's spiritual selves. In other words, they have used their physical challenge as a path to self-awareness.

In my years of working with and observing such people, I began to question some of the traditional psychological and medical approaches used in coping with major illnesses or injuries. I began to explore other methods of healing. Based on my own research and work, along with that of many other health care pioneers, I have come to the conclusion that it is time to enhance our current medical system by recognizing the emotional and spiritual factors that are crucial to good health.

We are now at a major turning point in medical history. We are discovering that the mechanistic approach to healing, which still holds power in helping to heal broken bones and combat certain infectious diseases, is not enough. Beyond this, we are seeing that there are emotional and spiritual components of healing whose power is considerable. When these are left out of medicine, as they have been in most modern medical approaches, even the benefits of the best that science has to offer are limited. To transform the mechanistic view through incorporating and infusing the spiritual and emotional components of healing is the task of this book.

The purpose of this book is to introduce the concept of transpersonal medicine. In it, I will discuss features outside the mechanistic view of health and disease, endeavoring to show that community support, love and prayer, the recognition of the sanctity of the human spirit, and a sense of connectedness to the life force are all powerful adjuncts to traditional methods of allopathic medical treatment. In addition, I will discuss practical applications—such as ritual, imagery, and altered states of consciousness—that harness the power of these energies.

WHAT IS TRANSPERSONAL MEDICINE?

Transpersonal medicine is a fundamental area of research, scholarship, and application based on people's experience of transcending their usual identification with their limited biological, historical, cultural, and personal selves and, at the most profound levels of experience possible, recognizing or even being "something" of vast intelligence and compassion that encompasses the entire universe. From this perspective our ordinary, normal, biological, historical, cultural, and personal self is seen as an important but quite partial (and often pathologically distorted) manifestation or expression of this much greater "something" that is our deeper origin and destination.

We are forced to use imprecise terms like *something*, because ordinary language, as a partial manifestation of our ordinary self, which is itself a partial manifestation of our deeper transpersonal "self," is of only partial use in our research and practice of transpersonal medicine, and needs to be supplemented with other expressive and communicative modalities. Transpersonal experiences generally have a profoundly transforming effect on the lives of those who experience them, both inspiring them with great love, compassion, and nonordinary kinds of intelligence—and also making them more aware of those distorting and pathological limitations of their ordinary selves that must be worked with and transformed to bring about full psychological and spiritual maturity. Because people ordinarily identify primarily with the personal, which tends to separate us, rather than with the transpersonal, which experientially impresses us with our fundamental unity with each other and all life, intelligent knowledge of the transpersonal can be of great potential value in solving the problems of a world divided against itself.

Jeanne Achterberg coined the term *transpersonal medicine* to bridge two major concepts. *Transpersonal* means "beyond the self," and *medicine* means "to make well."[1] The underlying principle of transpersonal medicine is that power in sources from beyond the self or beyond what we ordinarily consider consensual reality is available to be drawn upon and used to help heal ourselves and others. *Trans* denotes not only "beyond" (as in *transcendental*), but also "across" (as in *transfer*). It implies change or action. These three aspects of transpersonal process—the cross-personal, the extra- or *beyond*-personal, and the everchanging-personal—are all encompassed in the approach of transpersonal medicine.

In a larger sense, transpersonal medicine can be seen as an important outgrowth of the new consciousness evolving throughout the world, with its renewed respect for ancient methods that allow us to draw on broader realms of wisdom than the merely personal.

Examples of these broader realms can be seen in all spiritual traditions of healing, which universally acknowledge that there are three general paths toward wholeness—love, wisdom, and power. Love is about how we transform each other and ourselves through the bonds of relationship. Wisdom is a process of learning that is beyond knowledge and intelligence, the insight that sees interconnection among all aspects of existence. Power is not power over others, but rather the power to bring forth energies from oneself and others that have the potential to transform every level of our being.

At its foundation, transpersonal medicine draws on another ancient healing source: ritual. According to Jeanne Achterberg, ritual is "the universal foundation for all transpersonal medicine."[2] The true essence of ritual is the empowerment of an individual through the personal and collective use of symbols. A young man undergoes the rite of passage into adulthood in the bar mitzvah; a wedding ceremony or a graduation exercise grants a person new privileges and status. These are familiar rituals that mark turning points in people's lives, the *trans*- process. In each of them there is some homage paid to the power greater than ourselves—be it the community or a spiritual power beyond our individual identities. In them, the individual is given the hope and dream of success or the grace of love and forgiveness. A ritual articulates the ongoing connection between an individual and the universe so that the person knows that he or she is part of the fiber of life, a component and recipient of the love of God or supreme consciousness. The ritual serves as a reminder that everything and everyone has meaning.

Ritual takes us beyond the personal realm, to sources of support founded in the collective dynamic of others' intentions and relationships. It can tap into the power of love and energetic resonance which, as we will see, are important components of healing and change. The commitment and understanding of others taking part in a ritual can be of the greatest significance for the individual's transformational potential. The community spirit has a power of its own. The transpersonal therapist is aware of and sensitive to this power and uses ritual as a container in which potential collective resources can align themselves for the ultimate and necessary shifts toward health.

Group ritual processes can have the power of life and death, emotionally or physically. One well-known positive group ritual format can be seen in the meetings of Alcoholics Anonymous, acknowledged as a most successful treatment for alcoholism. In transpersonal medicine we are constantly discovering that through group ritual practice we each have access to extraordinary wisdom and knowledge that comes from sources beyond our personal intellects. We discover that we have the capacity to reach into our depths of understanding and find clarity and peace beyond what we might simply explain as "learning." We have found the rituals described later in the book to be a deep reservoir of love, wisdom, and power.

THE PRINCIPLES OF TRANSPERSONAL MEDICINE

Transpersonal medicine, as a concept and practice, has reemerged as a result of two major trends: (1) the frustration with the allopathic model of medicine, which has tried unsuccessfully to control the natural order by attempting to create a deathless or disease-free society; and (2) the lack of attention and respect given to the emotional and spiritual needs of people who are ill.

In allopathic medicine, health is defined as the lack of disease. What this definition fundamentally means is that a person's physical and mental faculties are functioning within a particular range that the medical system defines as "normal." If disease is present, allopathic medicine seeks its cause and treatment in external factors—a physical injury, an organic factor like bacteria, or a chemical factor such as a toxin, for example. Within transpersonal medicine, health is seen in terms that go beyond the mechanistic. Health is defined in more spiritual terms as balance or harmony within a person's body and in his or her relationship to the larger universe. If disease is present, transpersonal medicine would look beyond external factors, seeking deeper sources in *inner* factors.

Transpersonal medicine goes beyond the view of disease as merely a mechanical breakdown of some tissue or biochemical response, contained in a time and place. Instead, we look at disease and healing from an entirely different perspective that integrates larger emotional and spiritual factors. This new paradigm has a more complex view of disease, outlined in the following key points:

1. *Disease is a tear in the fabric of an individual's connection with the universe and community.* Rather than seeing disease simply as a malfunction of a body part, those involved in the transpersonal process regard disease as an integral part of personal development, an opportunity for growth and transformation. The transpersonal path of healing uses the meaning of the catastrophic event to reorient the patient's priorities and help him or her find or restore self-awareness, wisdom, and a sense of connection in the experience.

We grow from adversarial conditions, and our capacity to learn from them strengthens our character and our ability to care for others. Those who practice transpersonal medicine view disease as a learning process—a chance to learn important skills for coping with pain and suffering, an opportunity to explore the relationships between an individual and the community, and a possibility to experience the healing as a part of the relationship between the patient and the physician.

2. *Disease and health are viewed as lifetime processes.* Too often, a disease is seen to be contained in a time capsule: "I had measles when I was four" . . . "I got arthritis when I was fifty." Treatment has also

been placed in a time capsule: "I will be well in two weeks." From a transpersonal perspective of health and disease, time and space are disregarded as boundaries of causation.

Transpersonal medicine would hold that disease is a function of three components not bounded by time and/or space: spiritual development, cosmic connectedness, and evolution. Disease emerges as a bubble in this sea of underlying currents. It may manifest as encouragement for a necessary change or merely as a consequence of a past conflict. Transpersonal medicine assumes that health and disease are not limited in scope to time, yet continue to be important signs of the developmental process of the individual.

3. *Passion and joy are the best preventive medicine.* Today's concept of preventive medicine emphasizes denial and self-discipline. It operates on the assumption that one is doing something that promotes disease and that one has to stop doing it or get sick. There is no question that some habits—such as smoking or eating a diet high in fat—cause disease. Yet the single most predictable variable for many major diseases is the absence of joy and passion. For example, in research studies the primary criterion for the development of heart disease, back pain, and cancer appears to be a negative response to the simple question, "Are you happy?"[3]

One of the main therapeutic approaches in other cultures is dancing and singing, which are often connected to religious ritual. Successful health spas around the world build their programs around activities that spur joy and passion—music, art, exercise, writing. These forms can even be diagnostic approaches to unlock healing symbols and energies from the unconscious. My own work has brought me to the conclusion that the healing journey requires some venue for the experience of joy and passion. Without it, life becomes only a dead space in which the human spirit is eaten away and its life force destroyed.

4. *Disease can be equated with the breakdown of the relationship between body, mind, and spirit.* Unlike the present practice of defining disease in terms of measurable cellular dysfunction, the transpersonal approach includes ways to identify spiritual and emotional precursors to disease and to implement deeper healing as a result. These precursors include

internal factors such as loss of connectedness to others, loss of connectedness with a larger spiritual being, or loss of joy, passion, or hope. Many contemporary studies show that any one of these factors can be a precursor to a disease such as cancer, back pain, heart disease, chronic depression, premature aging, and compromised immune function.[4] In fact, the presence of any one of these internal factors is a more dependable predictor of eventual disease than any other "medical" measure found. Ironically, within modern medicine we can find no scientific justification for taking these factors seriously, even though statistical and clinical data show them to be accurate, consistent predictors of the course a disease takes.

Many other cultures have diagnoses that take some of the imbalances of body-mind-spirit into account. The most frequent diagnosis in my literature search has been "spirit-loss," a syndrome in which the person feels a sense of loss and meaninglessness instead of joy, passion, and purpose.

CONCLUSION: THE NEW MISSION IN HEALTH CARE

The need for a new paradigm of medical care is apparent. The ongoing research into the mysteries of human health (as opposed to rat health, upon which medical science now depends) deserves to be supported, yet the definition of true care must also be addressed. As the balances and resources of Mother Earth continue to be abused and used up, new diseases such as AIDS will continue to emerge and baffle the scientific world. We are losing the battle for both the quantity and quality of life and health.

As we search for the inherent meaning of the existence of humankind, questions arise: What does it mean to be human? to feel human? and to know what it is we need to become? Unless we can answer these questions, we cannot know what the meaning of health is, much less what healing is and what is to be accomplished by the process.

Transpersonal medicine is a set of concepts that address the very core of humankind, the personal as well as the collective evolution of human consciousness. It recognizes the self as unfolding through a progression of psychological and spiritual developments. It also regards the health of humankind as interconnected with the total life force, dependent on other animals, plants, and the elements. Even the stars and planets play some part in our sense of well-being.

Transpersonal medicine sees that health relies upon *balance*—the balance within ourselves as well as the balance in our relationships to each other and the rest of nature. This is hardly a new idea: our ancestors recognized these dimensions before our attitude toward nature shifted from one of equality to one of "master." Only with the dominance of the industrial age have we so completely regarded the natural world as ours to control or to manipulate for personal economic gain.

Finally, we are becoming more aware that another major evolution is taking place. We are seeing it in business, in families, in education, and certainly in health care systems. It is the evolution of human relationships, the new dimension of how we can better love and support each other. In medicine, it is manifesting in the space between us and the universe, the transpersonal space.

Transpersonal medicine offers opportunities to rediscover ageless approaches to healing as well as to integrate into them the discoveries of modern research. It invites us to a new understanding of the interactions of the body-mind-spirit universe. Some of the ideas presented in this book have been scientifically researched and documented in terms of their effective implementation, others are discussed in light of experiential validity, especially my own observations as a clinician. By scientific standards, the transpersonal medicine model is incomplete because it is rooted in respect for the mystery of life itself. No model will ever encompass the human spirit, for an individual or for a community. Perhaps the most important contribution of the transpersonal approach is that it takes us beyond the limits of measurable scientific data into the heart of the human mystery, inviting us to discover the deeper sources of healing: wisdom, power, and love.

This book is meant to embrace the mystery of healing, to embrace it as a fact of life, and to nurture our own sense of wonder about existence. There is no guarantee that any particular healing technique will be effective, largely because we do not have the capacity to understand the many planes and dimensions for the events of our lives. Yet it behooves us to appreciate those special times in which true understanding and spiritual change can occur.

||≡|||

Interview with Jim McQuade, M.D.

Psychiatrist, Clinical Cancer Center,
University of California, Irvine

Frank Lawlis: As a transpersonal psychiatrist working with chemical dependency and family issues, how does your approach differ from that of a conventional psychiatrist?

Jim McQuade: The techniques I use are not all that startlingly different from those of a conventionally oriented psychiatrist. I might use drawings, touch, or even ask about the spiritual practice of a patient, but the most significant difference is the context in which the therapy is set. When the work I do is set in a transpersonal context, the possibilities of healing are much greater than if we are just two separate human beings trying to relieve the suffering of one or both of us.

Within a transpersonal context, it is not just the patient who benefits; it is not just me who benefits; it is ultimately and hopefully the whole human species that benefits. Sometimes a session of therapy with a patient feels like the most significant thing we can do for the planet. Holding this attitude can raise the context of a therapy session to the sacred. In fact, I regard the work I do with my life, with others' lives, as sacred activity.

FL: Do you consider transpersonal therapy to encompass multiple realities?

JM: I was talking with a medical student who was very bright but was having trouble with medical school. He thought that becoming an anthropologist instead would meet all of his needs and there would be less suffering. He was a very spiritual person, and he talked about the difficulty of going through the discipline of the training process. I tried to interpret his situation in terms of service, explaining that if his aim were to get through life by minimizing the suffering he was going to have to deal with, he was always going to find himself in the wrong place. The level at which I work examines these questions: What is it we need to do to meet the suffering? How do we transform it as it transforms us?

On the process level, I realize that I could be talking about money or incest or drugs or illness. That is one reality. There are also emotional realities, and all these realities are encompassed on a spiritual level. It is like a great chain spiraling upward. I realize that everything is changing simultaneously, and I maintain that it is all enveloped in the spirit. As Matthew Fox said, "We are humans inside a soul, not a soul inside of a human being." Ultimately, working with ourselves and others is a spiritual undertaking. It is difficult to maintain that broad perspective, especially when someone is talking about having been raped. Yet I do my best work when I can keep the spiritual context in mind.

FL: In the "real" world, are there certain psychiatric diagnoses that are beyond the transpersonal realm of therapy?

JM: What I am trying to do is to cultivate a process of love, of understanding, and any psychiatric diagnosis can be worked with in that context. Depression is present at all levels—physical, emotional, and certainly spiritual. Dealing with addictions nearly always means addressing spiritual questions. In order to heal, the patients have to come to the conclusion that there is something larger than themselves, whatever that is. It does not necessarily mean they have to believe in God, but there must be something they consider more important than themselves. When we are restricted within the boundary of our bodies, we suffer.

FL: Do you think that drug addiction can actually be an expression of spiritual need?

JM: Recently someone asked me how to tell healthy from unhealthy spiritual paths. A genuine spiritual path connects us to our wholeness and our unity with others; unhealthy ones bring about a sense of separation. Many people have their first experience of oneness through drug use, sex, or spending money. They feel a dissolution of boundaries at that time, like a peak experience. A problem arises when they think that an external substance or experience is responsible for that feeling, and then they keep going back to it with that expectation. But the feeling does not return. The resulting experience of anxiety, urgency, and panic pushes the habit. A lot of people get out of the vicious circle by simply realizing that the external behaviors do not work. Addicts often say that they don't enjoy their drugs anymore, not because they don't have cravings anymore, but because the drugs are no longer fulfilling. They see through them. Instead of connection, they feel isolation and alienation again.

FL: Do you think that rehabilitation programs like AA work successfully at this level?

JM: Although I've never been through a twelve-step program, I have more and more respect for that process for a number of reasons. For example, the sponsor relationship is one that few people have experienced. It provides a person whose only basic purpose is to encourage the well-being in another person. So many people have missed that in their parenting or love relationships.

Unfortunately, in many of the twelve-step programs there is the need to identify someone who has "caused" the victim's pain. So much energy is caught up in that search. It is rarely acknowledged that those people who cause pain are usually in just as much pain as the victims, or more. Ultimately, if we could see that we are all in this boat together, that suffering and causing suffering are a result of projecting our shadow parts out, we could focus on spiritual renewal without having to blame someone else for our pain.

FL: That would require forgiveness.

JM: Forgiveness is certainly part of the process. It is a very difficult thing to do, and in part it is still a mystery to me. But even not being able to forgive is helpful in showing us where our attachments still remain and where we are stuck in our lives.

⫴ 2 ⫴

RITUALS

WHENEVER HUMAN BEINGS gather to ward off danger, to worship, or to acknowledge major changes, they develop rituals. These rituals honor life's transitions and passages, providing form, substance, and guidance in our lives. They often prescribe behavioral methods of dealing with important physical, social, and mental changes. As Jeanne Achterberg says, "Without rituals, we have no map for how to act, no occasion for people to share their common bonds and experiences."[1]

One of the primary themes throughout this book will be the ritual as a major feature of healing. Ritual provides a space in which the individual and the community can focus their intention, incorporating multiple dimensions of collective consciousness and invoking invisible forces for the sake of a person's well-being. In this chapter, I will focus on the group ritual process.

In 1984, I began to explore shamanic ritual as a process for promoting change and personal growth that embraces a belief in a higher truth, that is, a truth beyond our individual egos and personalities. Shamanic ritual is unique in that it offers ways to integrate spiritual with psychological and physical healing. From my perspective as a psychologist, it seemed that shamanic rituals could give shape and meaning to that aspect of human behavior we know as volition, or will, from which intention springs. It is intention that allows us to determine our own paths and change those paths when necessary for healing and personal growth.

Through the practice of ritual, intention becomes more tangible. Ritual allows us to step outside our normal lives, which are guided by complex, individualized habits of thinking, feeling, and acting. We can then gain new perspective on what we are doing and how we are living, which allows us to define ways to support changes we might desire. Since shamanic ritual is clearly directed to the inner world, it offers a more wholistic approach to human change than analytical methods that attempt to reduce the human experience to a medical model.

Another aspect of shamanism that appealed to me was that it views change as normal and sees all conflict as lessons on a spiritual, rather than material, life path. Within this system, the body is seen not as the be-all and end-all of our lives; rather, it is the vehicle for the spirit, which is not limited by time or space. A subtle but extremely important aspect of this vision is that the spirit is seen as ongoing, not limited to its present form, as attached to the body or the personality. Healing, or working with change on the individual level, has a higher purpose—to benefit the ongoing spirit of life on Earth. Thus, all our struggles—and their healing—have *meaning* beyond our individual selves. The purpose of healing has to do less with *adjustment* to painful situations, whatever they might be, than with changing in ways that bring peace and deeper insight.

I had been introduced to ritual and shamanism by Virginia Hine, noted social science pioneer, with whom I was associated for several years. Mrs. Hine's work provided much inspiration and guidance for the structured materials I present in the latter pages of this chapter.

I quickly discovered that, to understand shamanic ritual, one must experience it firsthand. And so it was that I began attending healing sessions by Native Americans in the Southwest, in order to learn directly from the masters of this tradition. In the summer of 1984, I found myself sitting in a "sweat lodge," a sort of airtight tent, heated with glowing rocks set in a pile at the center. Additional rocks were kept hot by a wood fire tended by an assistant outside the lodge; from time to time the supply of rocks in the lodge was replenished. The red-hot rocks were occasionally sprinkled with water, producing great quantities of steam that swirled all around us.

There were several people present. The shaman began by blessing the four directions—South, West, North, and East—praying to our ancestors for harmony and courage. Although the heat was intense, and sweat was pouring from our bodies, the circle of participants maintained a state of quiet reverence. The shaman was singing and beating a water drum. Though I did not know what his ancient songs meant, the essence of love and serenity that they conveyed struck a deep chord within me. The entire group seemed to move into a trance, temporarily suspended from all worldly concerns.

Before the sweat lodge began, one person from our group—we'll call him Curtis—had addressed the shaman and asked for a healing. Curtis described body pains he had been experiencing, including abdominal pain and difficulties sleeping and concentrating. The shaman listened for a while, receptive and empathetic. At times he requested more information about Curtis's family dynamics and medical background. When Curtis had finished telling his story, and the shaman had finished questioning him, he told Curtis to meditate while the rest of the group surrounded him with our support.

During the sweat lodge, Curtis was to symbolize the act of transition by taking a new name. When the rest of us left, Curtis was to remain in the sweat lodge until this new name came to him, emerging from his own consciousness. The new name would also help define a new mission for Curtis's life. So as not to distort this new mission, he was instructed to reveal this new name to no one. In the spirit world, however, he would be addressed only by this new name.

I do not know how long Curtis stayed in the sweat lodge after the rest of us had left, but when we came together again the next day, his face was filled with a new radiance. The symptoms of acute anxiety that he had described to us on the previous day were gone.

Curtis then told us how he had released childhood frustrations associated with being raised by an alcoholic mother. He had forgiven her for her human limitations. I asked if the heat of the lodge had somehow helped him to process this material more quickly than he might have in a more modern setting, for example, in the office of a psychotherapist. He answered that he felt that the whole process—the physical changes, the acts of communion, the focus on the inner life—had helped to take him into another realm of reality, allowing him to maintain a rather lengthy internal dialogue. I thought that the heat had probably altered Curtis's physiological balance, much as fasting or certain kinds of breathing exercises can do. This alteration had somehow enhanced a transition into other states of consciousness where change could be heightened and intensified.

The week after this experience in the sweat lodge, I was evaluating patients for orthopedic surgery, part of my job at that time. I decided to use some of the shamanic principles I had observed, this time applying them in a setting that was decidedly in the realm of Western medicine. It was my task as a psychologist to determine patients' states of anxiety and depression and to make recommendations concerning any problems these conditions might present for the patients while undergoing and recovering from complex surgery. Experience showed that patients who went into surgery in emotional turmoil tended to have more complications than those who went into treatment with positive expectations and relative calm. I was often asked to work with people in turmoil in order to help resolve conflicts so that treatment success was maximized and complications minimized. Resolving emotional problems also helped patients in rehabilitation.

On this particular day, I entered the room of a patient—we'll call him John. Though I'd never met John before, the moment I crossed the threshold, I knew that something extraordinary was about to happen. I did not know exactly what that would be.

Although I did not find him to be significantly depressed or anxious, John's medical prognosis was grim. X rays showed that he had an inoperable, fast-growing tumor wrapped around his spinal cord. Doctors felt that as the tumor grew larger John would experience increasing levels of pain, for which the medical staff could promise little or no relief. The doctors decided that John should remain in the hospital, with a private nurse at his bedside until his death, which they expected within a few days. He was coded for no life-support assistance if and when he went into a coma.

As a member of the pain-management team, I was to give both John and his wife support in the ordeal they would have to face. I felt that the situation called for a ritual, at least to honor the courage that the two of them would need in the days ahead. John's wife was particularly appreciative, welcoming the opportunity to participate in a positive way. The private nurse who'd been assigned to John was equally cooperative and enthusiastic about doing something constructive for the family. We decided to try holding the ritual whenever there was significant pain, or when any one of us would appreciate it. There was obvious affection throughout the group at this point.

I started the ritual by asking each person to express his or her spiritual beliefs. I asked them especially to discuss what time and space would mean within a person's body. Although each person had different views on these questions, all the views expressed were supported by the rest of us. At this point, we had entered into what I would later come to call the state of *awareness of universality*, the first stage of the subtle change of consciousness that ritual brings about.

Our next step was to join hands, close our eyes, and breathe together, joining in a kind of humming. In this way we were *severing* ourselves from our everyday realities, moving into a special place physiologically and psychologically. We were raising oxygen levels in our brains and bodies. We were also creating a special inner place for ourselves, embracing the beliefs and feelings unique to us at that moment. We were, in effect, entering our own "church," a place like the sweat lodge, where we could be in touch with our inner selves.

We all reached out and touched John with both hands, sending love and warmth toward him. Our only goal was that we might in this way bring about some constructive and comforting change. Such a change might help encourage a different self-concept, a different level of energy, a deeper form of relaxation, or a release from anything that might be troubling him.

As it turned out, it was not easy for John to receive this nurturing. Accepting support and emotional nourishment from others was an experience that he had never found comfortable in his long-term role as the father of a large family. He seemed ashamed to admit that he had reached a place in his life where he was helpless and needed others' support. After struggling with this feeling, he quickly learned how to put his shame behind him and receive the care and love offered him. He was able to open up to that energy, and as he did, John described what for him was a completely new experience—the experience of receiving love and affection without the belief that he would have to "pay it back." To him it was like discovering a sense of grace. This state is what I would later define as the *transitional* phase of ritual.

The fourth and final step for most rituals is the *return*—rejoining with the community—marked by some form of exchange or celebration to honor the completed process. In our completion of the transitional period, we exchanged our thoughts and feelings about the experience. As we repeated the ritual over the next few days, we would occasionally exchange small gifts, such as soft drinks or candy.

From the beginning, our goal had not been to *cure* John, nor was it our intent to challenge hospital procedures in any way. The fact is that staff nurses were very supportive of the ritual since they had no other way to manage the pain John would have to endure on the way to his impending death. My own goal was simply to increase John's tolerance for pain, since I knew that the kind of tumor he had could cause pain of the most horrible kind.

In spite of his grim medical prognosis, John did not die. He got better and better, healthier and healthier, his improvement noticeable even by the hour. A few days after the rituals began, John underwent another set of X rays, which showed that the tumor was in remission, shrinking at a rapid rate. Less than a week after the date that the medical staff had predicted for his death, John walked out of the hospital.

John's miraculous recovery encouraged me to explore further the power of ritual, increasingly introducing it into my work at the pain clinic. The results were dramatic. With one patient, a broken component of the bony structure of the vertebrae grew back into place within days. The healing ritual, originally intended only to bring relief from the pain she was suffering as a result of her spinal injury, also helped the patient resolve serious conflicts in her marriage. In another case, scar tissue that had caused chronic, debilitating pain dissolved. And in more cases than I can name, pain and suffering were greatly reduced, or at least made manageable, allowing people who had been totally or partially incapacitated to live normal, happy, and productive lives. Through ritual, we were also able to help people make significant psychological changes, such as emerging from severe depression, discovering new life missions, and opening up to new, more satisfying and productive relationships in their personal and professional lives.

THE HEALING PROCESS OF RITUAL

As used in transpersonal medicine, ritual reenacts in the outer world what is experienced in the invisible, imagistic world of visions and feeling. It enables people to transcend their self-boundaries, connecting with the power of hope and the consciousness of sacred space. But on a scientific basis, what do we know about the form of ritual that supports the supposition that these processes lead to any alteration of mental or physical conditions? Briefly, we discuss four areas of research that address the beneficial possibilities of ritual. From these, we can safely conclude that ritual reduces alienation, anxiety, and depression. Also, the studies support the concept that rituals can help activate transformative realities for necessary change and engage the power of transpersonal influence through what might be termed "energy" effects from others. These specific areas of interest are examined in more detail below.

Rituals Increase the Sense of Connectedness

A recent article in *Science* cited sixty-two studies that reveal strong supportive documentation that "lack of social support constitutes a major risk factor for mortality" and that social relationships protect health and enhance healing.[2] Social support was defined in a variety of ways, incuding marital relationships, friendships, general family relationships, group memberships, and relationships with health care professionals. The effects of these social support networks were seen to have consistent positive effects on such variables as surgical recovery time, likelihood of birth complications, birth weight, resistance to infectious diseases like tuberculosis, cardiovascular reactivity, ulcers, and general stress responses. Documented biochemical changes included increased growth hormones, lower cholesterol levels, enhanced white blood cell activity, and reduced sympathetic nervous activity.

We conducted a study with chronic and intractable back pain patients in a clinic in north Texas, in which variables were measured before and during a three-week stay in an inpatient ward. Included in the set of variables were a set of factors from the "Four Relationship Factor Questionnaire" that indicated the power of the bond the patients had with the therapy group in which they participated during their stay.[3] The factors measured were respect for the group's problem-solving abilities, identification with each other's problems, and ability to give affection when needed. Regardless of type of physical diagnosis, psychological profile, or treatment, the strength of the bond with the group was consistently the variable most connected with whether the pain was reduced or remained the same.

These studies support one aspect of the power of ritual—social connectedness, or universality. Ritual as a formal process provides at least a provision for the individual to receive these aspects of relationship in methods known from generations of healing, possibly influencing the deep spheres of consciousness beyond our immediate memories, and empowering the body-mind-spirit to harmony.

Rituals Encourage Hope

Inherent in reduced alienation is also a reduced sense of hopelessness. A broad array of research has demonstrated the correlated impact of hopelessness on a variety of psychological and physical dysfunctions, including cancer growth and gastrointestinal conditions.[4] Prolonged stress has long been held to impede healing through the sustained arousal of biochemical factors such as certain hormones, setting the stage for the diagnosed conditions of cardiovascular and immunity deficient diseases that result from a compromised resistance to invasion.[5] More important for chronic conditions, stress has been listed as a probable agent in the decrease of damaged cell recovery through a mechanism of the DNA repair process. The argument that stress has a negative influence upon both psychological and physical processes has been articulated and incorporated into the general context for health care.

Conversely, the role of stress reduction in health care is more indirect in terms of evidence. We can extrapolate from the biochemistry of stress the assumption that the reduction of stress would enhance health, at least to the point of negating the destruction created by anxiety and depression. If ritual can help create self-esteem and relaxation, it follows that the corticosteroids and vasoconstriction related to both catecholamines and muscular tension would decrease. As stress is reduced, the hyperactive hormones and body tension could be restored to balance. Because biofeedback treatment focuses on the patient's ability to relax the body and mind, many diseases and symptoms, such as hypertension and tension headaches, resolve themselves through training. These methods are considered treatment of choice for many disorders that are stress-induced because they educate the patient to control his or her symptoms.

One of the pioneering studies in this field was conducted by Peavey, Lawlis, and Govern to test the hypothesis of enhanced health through stress-management process.[6] They divided a group of college students into high- and low-stressed subgroups and evaluated their respective immunity factors, principally the neutrophils' response. (Neutrophils are white blood cells that constantly patrol one's bloodstream for toxins and other "enemies.") As expected, achieving results later replicated in several studies, the high-stressed participants were significantly more impaired in terms of immunity factors than the low-stressed group. The study offered the next step in which the high-stress subjcts participated in a stress-management program. An evaluation afterward revealed that the high-stress participants' immune responses had changed to approximate that of the low-stress participants.

In a recent article published in the *Clinical Psychology Review* evaluating the implications of stress management specifically for postsurgical issues, 168 references were cited.[7] The conclusion of the article was that the most fruitful approach was to target the ritualistic features of the hospital ward for positive attribution in surgical procedures. More specifically, it suggested social support and opportunities for active coping for direct enhancement of physiological features.

Lawlis, Selby, Hinnant, and McCoy conducted a well-controlled retrospective study in which specific ritual-related features (anxiety-reduction skills, consciousness-altering techniques, and family support instructions) were administered to patients undergoing immediate back surgery.[8] The results were indicative of improved healing processes by significantly shorter hospital stays, as well as fewer pain indicators and fewer complications. The most consistent finding has been that psychological approaches, regardless of orientation, do help patients in terms of increasing hopefulness and reducing anxiety or depression.

Rituals Extend Influence beyond the Normal Psychobiological Influence

The concept of enhancing health by strengthening interpersonal supportive relationships and stress management is now widely accepted. Researchers Larry Dossey and William Braud have taken this concept a step further in studies that suggest that the influence of *intention*—a primary component in ritual—has a direct bearing on health and healing. While this influence may be accounted for in human consciousness models, it cannot be totally accounted for in current scientific models of energy exchange nor by individual differences. The major discussion of these models will be examined more thoroughly in a chapter on the nonlocal mind and the possibility of interaction between two individuals from a distance. However, because the impact of external influence from a group of caring people upon the psychological and physical aspects of a body is obviously relevant to ritual, I will discuss it here. This aspect would certainly be truly "transpersonal."

In similar methodology to that used by LeShan, in the pain clinics that I codirected I conducted many experiments in the occurrence of physiological changes in individuals from the distant influences of groups.[9] Between ten and fifteen patients admitted for the treatment of chronic pain participated in each study group. In each experiment, one member of the group was selected as the focus patient. The focus patient would then leave the group and go into a separate room, where he or she was hooked up to biofeedback equipment to measure psychological and physical responses. At random times, and unbeknownst to the subject, the prayer group would focus on the patient, sending him or her their love and support. At these times, the biofeedback machines measured an elevated skin temperature, indicating a physical change in the subject, and an increased sense of well-being, indicating a psychological change.

Research helps objectify our clinical perceptions; however, what was not documentable were the number of extraordinary changes that occurred partially by design and partially as a critically desired event for rehabilitation. For patients suffering from the pain of scar tissue around the nerves of the spine, the rehabilitation is difficult due to the discomfort from the process of stretching and gradual change required for some release of the tissue. For many weeks, patients have to do exercises that stretch the scar tissue and nerves on a consistent basis. The process is problematic because of the occasional spasms and tears that occur as results of the therapy. I have come to the conclusion that unless patients can learn, by shifting their consciousness, to transcend the pain, it is almost impossible to withstand the therapy. Unless the patients undergo some change in self-concept and realize the pain as somehow relevant to their lives, the process is not endurable.

When the patients were discharged from the hospital, the exit interview would always request information about what they remembered as being the most positive, the most negative, the most therapeutic, and other similar aspects of their experiences. Among the successful patients, the consistent description of the most important and unforgettable experience was the "love" they felt from the staff and patient groups. In fact, when asked to articulate what the central elements of their rehabilitation programs were, most (90%) could not describe them in concrete terms, such as "changing behavior patterns," or "learning new exercise patterns." Almost to a person, they would discuss some magical moment when they felt a strong wave of love that helped them through the discomfort and discouragement. Some could define it as a spiritual experience, while others would relate the feeling to being in a natural family where people "really cared." However love is defined, it is at least expressed through some altruistic energy intending the well-being of another person. Anecdotal evidence is extremely pervasive with regard to the healing power of love within the community context.

Ritual Can Create Conditions Necessary for Transformation

It is within the context of ritual that transformation can occur most easily. As Richard Moss remarked in *The I That Is We*, it is through the community process that we can most effectively achieve transformation. He also predicted that the future of healing lay almost totally within groups and communities.

The integration process of transformation is extremely difficult without ritual. To change one's life requires tremendous courage, and to have this change honored and respected by those around one is critical. All research comparing individual and group psychotherapy supports this conclusion.

Rituals are used to honor a person's transition from one state to another. Without ritual there is no specific time or place where one can pinpoint the change, and there is no overt respect given to a person's new role. The lifestyle that enhanced the disease state must die in order for the person to reestablish a state of harmony and health. For example, the person with a diagnosis of alcoholism must change; however, to change independently within the context of a community is difficult because of expectations and role development. The strength of the habit that the body and mind have created is reinforced by external forces. It is the alcoholic whose life is required to change; however, the problem of alcoholism is a community and family problem. Again, the principles underlying the rehabilitation experienced in AA are ritualistic in nature. "Rituals for healing have the purpose of giving credence and significance to life transitions; they provide maps of form for guidance during perilous times when bodies, minds, and spirits are broken. The acts of ritual allow people to share their common experiences and to give visible support to each other. The symbols and events of healing ritual cement the healer/healee bonds and engender faith and hope that the passage into the place of wholeness, harmony, or relief of suffering will be achieved."[10]

The Shape of Ritual

Over years of studying rituals from a wide variety of cultures, I have noticed a fourfold pattern to ritual that seems universal. This pattern is what makes shamanic ritual particularly valuable for accomplishing the kinds of life changes I discuss in this book. Though the four key steps are known by many different names, depending on the tradition from which they spring, their functions are remarkably alike. In my own work, I have found it helpful to name them according to function: (1) *awakening* to the awareness of universality, (2) *severance* from everyday reality, (3) *transition* into a new personal identity, and (4) *return* to one's everyday reality. The shortened versions, in italics above, are used for convenience.

1. *Awareness of universality.* Throughout history, societies have used art, music, science, and religion to express that we are all part of a larger whole. There are parts of the human experience that we all share, a continuum in which each of us participates that is much larger than any one of our lives. In the first part of the ritual, the individual acknowledges that there is a past and a future, stretching off in infinite directions from the present, and that there is a reality, perhaps including an intelligence much larger than our individual identity, of which we are an integral part.

The awareness of one's universality need not have a religious, or even a spiritual context. It may or may not be derived from an existing dogma. People might observe their part in a continuum in any number of ways—from an awareness of carrying an ongoing bloodline, to acknowledgment that one's own life touches others in important ways that cannot be defined or judged, and even to the feeling that we are all part of an ongoing exchange of constantly recycling atomic particles.

The important thing about this part of the ritual is acknowledging that whatever our lives represent, and whatever circumstances we have experienced or are now experiencing, our experiences may have a universal meaning or purpose that is not necessarily ours to comprehend. It is interesting to note here that this part of the ritual is expressed in the first step of the popular twelve-step recovery programs, wherein the individual admits to a need for strength, guidance, and support from a power greater than him- or herself.

2. *Severance*. In most ritual, the individuals are taken out of the context of their daily lives. This severance can be real or symbolic and usually involves the persons' being removed from their normal daily contacts, the usual ways they have of relating to the people and circumstances in their lives. To the extent that it is possible, the individuals are temporarily relieved of all their ordinary responsibilities, duties, and privileges. This can be achieved by physiological, psychological, or geographic separation from their everyday lives.

3. *Transition*. This phase of ritual is often called "liminal," from the Latin word meaning "threshold." It implies a process of entering a place, or state of being, that is different from anything that one has ever before or will hereafter experience. In the transition phase, we experience life in an other-than-ordinary way. This phase might involve undergoing a test or ordeal, encountering images that evoke the past or future, meeting fantasy figures that take us "out of ourselves"— all so that we might undergo our own ritual death and rebirth. In the process, we are put in touch with spiritual sources of power that we may or may not have known were available to us. As a result, our previous sense of personal identity is broadened and permanently altered.

The transitional phase is usually characterized by a degree of chaos and upheaval. We saw this in the story about John's recovery from cancer: his habitual inability to receive comfort and support from others had to fall away before he could open to the help that was coming to him. We are provided with the support necessary to endure this period of upheaval and change by participating in the ritual with others who are undergoing similar life changes. The initiates interact as equals, shorn of all previous status—naked, defenseless, and vulnerable.

4. *Return*. This fourth phase of ritual is, classically, the actual return of the persons to the community from which they came. There, ideally, the individuals find both recognition that they have changed and support for the change, allowing them to integrate with their external, everyday lives what has happened to them internally during the first three phases of the ritual. Persons return to the community changed, in effect different people, and the community, in turn, treats them

differently, acknowledging and supporting them in their new identity. Because of the changes, individuals are given roles in the community that make full use of who they are now. This means assuming new responsibilities, gaining new privileges, and functioning in a different way than before the ritual. There is a symbolic emphasis on welcoming the persons back into the community and valuing them in ways that are commensurate with their changes.

In integrating the above four-step process with modern life, it may be helpful to look at how these steps might manifest in our own society. Perhaps the most graphic example is a young person's induction into the armed services. The induction begins with the new recruits being made aware of their part in the defense of the country. The big picture presented at that time is that each individual is dependent on every other, and every person must serve a common purpose (defense) without regard to his or her ego or personal needs. This would represent the *awareness of universality* stage.

The inductees are taken away from home, community, and loved ones, in short, removed from all familiar landmarks and social roles that once helped them define their personal identity. This, clearly, is the *severance* stage of the ritual, and is probably most dramatically symbolized in shaving the male inductees' heads, thus removing an important semblance of personal identity.

After the severance from the old identity, the inductees begin living with others like themselves in a camp that isolates them from what they have previously known. Now they are in the *transition* phase. They are given new clothes to wear and enter a rigorous training that requires them to live in a brand-new way. There are new rules of behavior, new foods, and a complete restructuring of how they spend their time.

Eventually, in most cases, the inductees adopt their new role, becoming soldiers, and once again participate in the larger society which, in turn, supports and values them in their new identity. This last phase is, of course, the *return*.

Two Kinds of Ritual

Anthropologists divide rituals into two types: (1) rites of passage, and (2) rites of intensification. Rites of passage are ceremonies that mark a life transition, or crisis. Examples of these include from nonbeing to being (birth), from childhood to adulthood, from bachelorhood to marriage, from illness to health, and from life to death. Baptism, bar mitzvahs, weddings, and funerals are rituals in our society that mark rites of passage.

Rites of intensification are intended to reinforce social bonds, to renew commitments to family or community, and to resolve conflicts with individuals or groups. Examples of these in modern society include national holidays, the celebration of our birthdays, and of course reaffirmations of one's religious beliefs during holidays like Hanukkah or Christmas.

But the fact of the matter is that there is a dearth of meaningful ritual in our culture, in the healing arts and elsewhere. Throughout history, ritual has nurtured the human spirit. But with the emergence of the scientific age, anything that could not easily be quantified, or "proven according to the scientific method," tended to be relegated to the category of "meaningless superstition." The human spirit, the "inner life," and all the ways we once had of nurturing that part of our being thus tended to be discarded. In part, we have lost meaningful rituals because we have lost our respect for the process of ritual. Thus, in some ways, the rituals we still observe are mere relics—hollow remnants of older, more genuinely experienced, more meaningful celebrations.

William Bridges, who writes brilliantly on human development, in *Transitions*, writes:

> People sometimes bewail the fact that we lack rituals and suggest that we ought to create some. Clearly the rites of passage were terribly important ways of validating and facilitating development. But our own situation cannot be remedied by rituals when we have lost our understanding of what rituals dramatize. Before rituals can have any real meaning for us, we must recover our understanding of, respect for, and willingness to experience the process of death, liminality, and renewal. For all of us have natural cycles of regeneration, though each of them requires a little death, a small winter, a subtle

crucifixion. I don't suppose we can recapture the primeval rhythm in our society at large, but individually and in small groups we can.[11]

What Bridges calls "death, liminality, and renewal" corresponds to the three stages of *severance, transition,* and *return* that I have described.

CREATING A RITUAL

Ritual can be defined as a series of archetypal acts using a set of symbolic objects. There are a few archetypal acts that have been used to symbolize severance, transition, and return in so many different cultures across space and time that they elicit responses in even the most ritually untutored heart. The three lists on page 33 may be used as a springboard in generating our own rituals or in helping others generate theirs.

Symbols

The capacity to use symbols is not only inherent in human nature, it is what many scholars use as the hallmark of humanness. It is natural and easy for most people to choose objects with symbolic meaning for them for use in creating their own rituals. The following ideas might also be helpful.

First, a symbol is more than an object that *represents* something else. A symbol connects the definable with the indefinable, the manifest with the unmanifest, the microcosm with the macrocosm. It points beyond what it represents. All symbol systems, writes Joseph Campbell, "function simultaneously on three levels: the corporeal of waking consciousness, the spiritual of dream, and the ineffable of the absolutely unknowable."[12]

The power of traditional symbols lies in shared meaning with which a group has invested an object. The larger the group and the more unquestioningly they believe in the reality behind the symbol, the more power it has to affect social and physical reality. Now that we know what we do about mind/body interpenetration and the power of

ARCHETYPAL ACTS

Severance	Transition	Return
Procession to a sacred area	Touching sacred objects	Leaving sacred area
Crossing a threshold	Isolation	Recrossing a threshold
Leaving the familiar	Vigils	Reentry into the familiar
Setting aside symbols of status/role	Living in communities without status/role	Accepting symbols of new status/role
Removing symbolic clothing	Nakedness	Donning symbolic clothing
Cutting hair	Changing hairstyle	Exchanging cut hair
Knocking down, smashing, breaking	Mutilating body	Mingling blood
Cutting, burning	Changing name	Building up
Tearing, burying	Lifting up, raising high	Exchanging gifts
Eating, drinking	Fasting	Fusing, joining objects
Untying, washing off	Ordeals, stress, tests, making vows	Tying, knotting
Veiling	Keeping silent	Sharing
Lighting candles or lights	Being immersed in water	Feasting
Stripping away	Keeping celibate	Sharing pipes, smoke
Purification	Altering consciousness	Handclasps, embrace
	Enacting change	Unveiling
	Dying and being reborn (symbolically)	Taking lights from common source
	Experiencing liminal state with co-initiates in unfamiliar or dangerous conditions	Making a circle
		Group chanting, singing

consensus, it is easier to understand the healing power of a quartz crystal, a cross, or chicken feathers or sand designs.

In medical settings we find the symbolic use of aspects of treatment highly significant. For example, when I was the consulting psychologist on the kidney dialysis unit in San Antonio, I attempted to make the patients feel more relaxed by wearing regular street clothes on the ward. However, many patients complained that they felt I was not really helping them unless I was wearing a white lab coat. Once I began to wear my lab coat, there was an immediate positive result. Whether it is the white coat of the healer, the magic smell of the soup, or the color of the pill, the symbol of healing must be recognized and embraced in order to enhance the healing potential of any treatment.

There are many self-generated rituals in which personal symbols are useful. Their effectiveness depends on the energy that goes into selecting them. Anything, either natural or manmade, can be a meaningful symbol. Shapes, colors, numbers, and directions all have important, though different, symbolic meaning in every culture. Some strike deep into archetypal levels of human experience. The cross, for example, is not peculiarly Christian. It is found in some form in almost every symbol system including that of the Kalahari Bushmen, who have been painting it in their sacred caves since prehistorical times. The numbers three and four are particularly important universally. The colors with the longest history of symbolic use are white, black, red, and yellow because Mother Earth made them so widely available to paleolithic peoples in clays, charcoal, iron- and ochre-bearing rocks. For those interested in exploring the cross-cultural or historical meanings of symbols, J. E. Cirlot's *Dictionary of Symbols* is useful.

Tools for Ritual

There are a few tools that can be helpful in planning a ritual. I have categorized these according to various components of ritual to provide a framework of choice. Drawn from a variety of anthropological sources, this list is at least suggestive, if not complete. (The components were prepared and circulated by Virginia Hine.) No ritual utilizes all of the components, but most include more than one.

- *Music:* from simple drumming to bells and/or trumpets, recorded or live; singing or chanting
- *Dancing and physical movement:* endless shuffling in a circle; swaying; rhythmic walking; mind-altering Sufi dancing; positioning individuals or groups to symbolize roles, relationships; moving to symbolize changes

- *Incantation and prayer:* addressing a deity, a common source of light or energy, the spirit of a heroic figure, the "Buddha within"; calling into awareness the "higher self" or higher power; formal prayer, drawn from traditional sources chosen in advance by participants; informal, spontaneous prayer; conscious use of the power in consensus
- *Statement of beliefs:* sermons, creeds repeated, myths retold, readings from scriptural texts, poems specially chosen or written
- *Mimetic acts:* use of effigies; enacting in pantomime or dance a desired outcome; dramatic reenactment of myths, legends, symbolic stories
- *Use of mana power:* transfer of power or energy through touch; touching a sacred or totemic object; laying on of hands, "tuning in" in a circle; ritual embrace; wearing sacred objects
- *Taboo:* abstention for ritual purposes—including silence, fasting, celibacy; taboos against touching or interaction, abstaining from normal relationships
- *Stress induction:* inducing physiological states designed to affect mental-emotional-spiritual states; ordeals, labors, and vigils, including vision quests; sensory deprivation; pain ritually inflicted; fatigue; hunger, thirst, sleeplessness
- *Vows:* taking a vow in front of others, often combined with shared food or an act of symbolic sacrifice
- *Feasting:* sharing sacred or symbolic food and drink, often combined with vows
- *Offerings:* making animal, food, or human sacrifice; making offerings of any sort, including burning incense or other dried plant material to stimulate the olfactory sense or to purify; offering smoke as a conduit for the divine
- *Congregation:* witnessing; processing, participating
- *Induction of altered or mystic states of consciousness:* meditating; chanting, dancing, or drumming; ingesting drugs according to a ritual pattern
- *Site selection:* choosing place for symbolic reasons; setting

aside a place as permanent sacred space; preparing an area
for temporary use as sacred

WHAT RITUAL CAN ACCOMPLISH

It is my belief that some of the drug problems we presently face in our
society derive, at least in part, from our search for spiritual meaning.
We can trace this back to the 1960s when hallucinogenic drugs such as
LSD seemed to offer insights that were once accessed only through
ritual and a long, rigorous education in spiritual values. In this respect,
drugs served a longing that was, more often than not, poorly defined,
poorly understood, and seldom discussed in respectable society. Divorced from true understanding, drugs were used, consciously or unconsciously, in an attempt to satisfy a human need that simply could
not be satisfied so easily.

With the revolution in consciousness that started in the 1960s, however, there has come an increased awareness of the needs of the human
spirit as well as an increased conviction that the so-called intangibles
of the human experience are vitally important. Interestingly, it was
science that helped us find our way back to the powers as well as the
needs of the human spirit. For example, through quantum physics we
learned that the mere presence of an observer alters that which is observed. Human consciousness, far from being intangible, interacts with
physical reality, altering its very nature. In our quest to understand
external reality, we have once again been forced to look inward as
much as outward. As Saint Francis of Assisi reflected nearly eight hundred years ago, "What we are looking for is what is looking."

Through my experience as a psychologist working within the medical community, it has become increasingly clear to me that our physical
health mirrors our psychological, spiritual, and interpersonal lives. In
working with patients facing severe chronic pain and imminent death,
it has become clear that through the human consciousness we can
bring relief, comfort, and even healing that even the greatest advances
in medical science cannot yet offer. Shamanic ritual provides us with
the framework for integrating the spiritual with changes that might
otherwise include only the physical and psychological.

Depending on who is performing it and how it is being performed, ritual can be a truly transformational experience, altering the way the participants live their lives from that day forward. Ritual serves many purposes and can accomplish a variety of functions. It can help us move from ordinary to nonordinary levels of consciousness, even bridging multiple levels of consciousness simultaneously. It can help us get in touch with the wisdom and energy contained in archetypal situations, characters, and actions, opening us more fully to what C. G. Jung called the "collective unconscious." Through ritual, we can gain access to our own inherent powers and gifts, renewing and regenerating our energies. Ritual also allows us to transcend habitual beliefs and per- spectives, including self-perceptions and attitudes toward our own lives. A ritual might help us to reaffirm our commitment to a belief, relationship, or personal goal, or affirm a feeling that we wish to carry into action. It gives us a venue for participating in myths that can nur- ture us, guide us, and help us grow. Through ritual we can give form to "intangibles" of human life, making them deeper and more mean- ingful. We can renew bonds with our community, tune in to nature, and open ourselves to participation in the workings of the universe.

When we look at what works, at what it is that triggers the processes necessary to restore health through the human consciousness, ritual stands out as an unrivaled tool. When we look beneath the surface, we discover that ritual works not because of some hidden mystical quality but because it fosters change through bringing to consciousness a vi- sion of a higher truth, an aspect of ourselves that both encompasses and transcends individuality.

Interview with Barbara Dossey, R.N., M.S.

Author of *Critical Care Nursing: Body, Mind, and Spirit* and *Rituals in Medicine*

Frank Lawlis: How do you regard ritual in medicine, especially on the level of consciousness?

Barbara Dossey: What is important is the difference between a routine and a ritual. For example, in working on my book on rituals, the copyeditor became confused and asked, "Are you just giving relaxation a new name?" Imagery and relaxation are components of the process, but what we are trying to do is expand consciousness. That is what happens in ritual. We are looking at how one can really expand consciousness, where one can look at health from the perspective of expanded consciousness. We are looking at how physiology and consciousness can come together.

When we talk about "transpersonal," we are talking about people going beyond their personal uniqueness into a deep connection with others, the earth, and the cosmos. Ritual may begin with a simple skill, but it takes one to a new level of awareness where wholeness can be seen in the context of a process. Ritual is a process in which one begins to take a cultural belief or value one has through a series of transforming events, thereby deepening one's sense of consciousness and empowerment. Something happens when one enters a sacred space and finds a core of transpersonal connectedness. One finds the invisible force for change and healing there. Whether it lasts for fifteen minutes or fifty minutes, it creates a period of transition.

FL: When you mention the entering state, are you referring to what we call an altered state of consciousness?

BD: That is a good way to describe it. What happens is that we come to a new understanding of what it means to be present, present with self and present with others. We come to a state in which our day-to-day perception of things is different. We find ourselves opening to new things in a new space from which we can get in touch with oneness at a universal level.

FL: When you use the word *new* two images emerge for me. One is a change in reality, and the second involves creativity.

BD: Both processes happen, especially in terms of creativity. When we talk about creativity, the most important thing is that in being present with ourselves, we can allow body and mind to enter into a quiet space where the intention is to connect with a healing state. In that state we can affirm our wholeness, which allows us to open up a sensitive and creative way of looking at ourselves.

What is presence about? What is it that takes us so far from that core of presence? How do we get back into it? Breathing exercises are very helpful in touching in with that space. Breath is like a loop of awareness one can use to get in touch with oneself. Once a patient gets that going, the therapist can pace his or her breath with the patient's, and true presence can come about between two individuals. They can come together into the same space, into presence.

Ego wants intellectual answers to the questions, "Who?" "What?" "When?" "Why?" What happens when we become fully present is that we give space to our feelings of connectedness. When we become present, judgment gives way to nonjudgment, and we are able to return to the moment with intention. That is how healing happens.

Ritual is a space in which we can return to intention and presence. What you do is not as important as your purpose, your basic goal, your motivation. What is your truest and clearest hope? That can be the ground for healing.

FL: When you train nurses, what do you tell them to do in their work in regard to rituals or consciousness change?

BD: First the nurses have to change their own state of consciousness if they want to work on that level with others. For example, every time nurses do an intake interview, they can create a sacred space for that task. They can enter a state of mind in which they are truly listening to the information the patient is giving them as a story. By doing this we can rediscover the healing in our practice and have a new relationship with the patient, with the uniqueness of each person. We can begin to connect with that person because much of their story will reflect much of ours.

Recently I had a reunion with some old girlfriends. All of our lives have been so different—different professions, different experiences. It was a wonderful time to talk about my life. I began to realize that this also could be the experience of a patient on an intake interview; it could be the opportunity to tell their story and maybe to learn something about themselves. It could be a healing experience. It was for me. Every time we take an intake interview, we can connect genuinely with another human being.

For example, in taking the history of a patient with pain, you can begin to hear the echoes of self, the patterns of self-perceptions as common themes occur. You may have heard the history of the pain of myocardial infarction many times, but you have not heard this individual's experience of it. In listening to the cultural metaphors, the imagery and the symbols, you can look for themes. Sports come up frequently, "I am winning with this disease." "I am being coached in this." Machine metaphors are also common: "The pump is bad." If we can begin to bring magic, the sacred, into the work by connecting with the patient on this level, the world of nursing will be the mission we wanted.

The other thing I try to teach nurses is to get out of the way of the patient's healing. Too often when we learn of a disease, we want to fix it, to tell the patient what to do. When I was working in the biofeedback lab, I would find myself telling patients to relax, which of course did not help them relax. I had to learn to get out of the way, to respect the patient's journey, because that is the most important thing anyway.

A third aspect of my work with nurses involves encouraging them to redirect their attitude about work, encouraging them to listen to their colleagues talk about their patients, and to begin to listen for the metaphors they use when doing so. It brings communication to a higher level. Then when the nurse goes to the bedside of the patient, he or she can be present much more immediately. The important thing is to listen to the stories in a new, open way, which brings it all together, for the team and the patient. It does not make any differences how good our medical science is unless we can also enhance the patient's own internal healing process. It is a privilege to listen and understand, to support the patient and each other.

‖‖ 3 ‖‖

TRANSPERSONAL
IMAGERY AND
HEALING

O NE OF THE MAJOR principles of transpersonal psychology is the
general assumption that consciousness has no boundaries. The
influence of one person's thoughts can and probably does have an
impact upon others. In the sense that we as individuals are parts of a
greater whole, the notion that we are separated by time and space is
only an illusion. Consciousness may be a field, like that of gravity or
electromagnetism, that enhances a bond of communication that may
or may not be manifest within our limited range of sensitivities and
perception.

This general theory of "one mind" consciousness is similar to the
"hundredth monkey" myth. This is the story of an island that was
populated with thousands of monkeys whose primary food source was
destroyed by poor weather conditions. Researchers began to drop potatoes to them, but the monkeys, having never eaten potatoes, did not
know what to do with them. Finally a monkey discovered how to wash
and eat one, and began to teach the others. As the hundredth monkey
was taught, all the rest of the monkey population began to know how

42

to eat potatoes without being taught. This story illustrates the idea that knowledge can permeate a community without the process of individual learning. This concept explains how we may have cumulative knowledge from our ancestors as well as from those now around us. The coincidences of inventions and discoveries made within minutes or days of each other, even at different places on earth, would be explainable by this theory.

The great paleoanthropologist Pierre Teilhard de Chardin taught that consciousness permeates all of matter, from lowly rocks to human beings. There now appears to be growing evidence to support his views. For example, the work of Cleve Backster seems to suggest that plants can react to emotional situations (watering, burning of a leaf, "watching" brine shrimp being dumped into boiling water) and even to the unspoken intentions of the experimenter.[1]

Larry Dossey, in *Recovery of the Soul*, has postulated an awareness of this principle of no-boundary consciousness in medical terms. In his definition of Era III medicine, he concludes that some healing may be influenced by factors not in direct association with the patient. He has categorized as Era I medicine the paradigm that maintains that the body is composed of discrete systems/organs whose functioning is deterministic in nature, as was the clockwork universe of the Newtonian physics on which it was based. In this paradigm, the effects of mind and consciousness are regarded as inconsequential, and all medical interventions are physical and external—drugs, surgery, radiation. Era II medicine encompasses an awareness of the mind-body relationship, acknowledging that emotions and attitudes affect the human body. For example, the role of stress has been almost universally accepted as a major factor in today's most frequent diseases, including heart attacks, strokes, and hypertension; behavioral medicine is now generally recognized as a professional specialty within medical schools. Era III medicine recognizes that consciousness is both nonlocal (therefore capable of acting and being acted upon from a distance) and nontemporal (not confined to a past-present-future cause-and-effect model).

In his theory of relativity, Einstein showed that time is not the absolute it had been thought to be. As objects approach the speed of light, time shrinks to zero. The theory of black holes in space postulates that time may even reverse itself. The issue of space and cause-effect has also been challenged by Bell's Theorem, which has been tested in physics laboratories, which states that the impact of one proton spin can influence the spin on another proton if those two protons had some earlier encounter, even though each may be on an opposite side of the universe. The implications for interactions between humans, as collections of protons and atoms, have been extrapolated to explain how interaction between people can occur even when they are in different parts of the world.

Three of the most prestigious scientists of the twentieth century subscribed to unconventional notions of nonlocality of consciousness. Physicist Erwin Schrödinger, mathematician-logician Kurt Gödel, and Albert Einstein all believed in a "one mind" theory of which each person is a part. Helmut Schmidt theorizes that no two minds are separate or discrete entities, but are interconnected and omniscient, instances of a holographic reality.[2] This interconnectedness is the foundation of the explanation given by many healers for how healing influences move from one individual to another. It is also the premise on which the power of negative processes such as hexes and curses is based.

HEALING THROUGH TRANSPERSONAL SPACE

Healers have been active at least since the beginnings of recorded history. The literature of medical anthropology as well as cross-cultural studies show that virtually all non-Western societies and most of the non-Anglo communities in the United States still use some form of indigenous healing that lies outside the realm of traditional allopathic medicine.[3] The fact that the art of healing has been in existence for so long attests to the underlying belief that healers have special abilities to use their consciousness to help others. If one could assume that belief has to have at least some validity to exist, then one would have to accept that the art of healing is a phenomenon worthy of investigation and recognition.

According to Merriam-Webster's *Ninth New Collegiate Dictionary*, the word *heal* comes from the Middle English *helen* and the Old

English *hal*, meaning "whole." The first two definitions given are "to make sound or whole," and "to restore to health." Healing has also been defined as "the intentional influence of one or more persons upon another living system without utilizing known means of intervention."[4] Types of healing include psychic, mental, faith, paranormal, native, and shamanic. Many techniques are practiced: healing from a distance, passing hands near the body or touching the person, meditating for the person to be healed. All the types and techniques seem to involve a special state of mind that creates a feeling of oneness with the healee and the cosmos.

Nowhere is the process of healing more documented than in reports of the activities of Jesus Christ. For example, in Matthew 8, verses 5–6 and 13, we read:

> And when Jesus was entered in Capernaum, there came unto him a centurion, beseeching him and saying, "Lord, my servant lieth at home sick of the palsy, grievously tormented." And Jesus said unto him, "I will come and heal him." . . . And unto the centurion, "Go thy way and as thou hast believed, so be it done unto thee." And his servant was healed in the self-same hour.

Many healers have been studied in recent years, with interesting and impressive results. Rafael Toledo, a physician specializing in pediatric cardiology in Texas and a member of the behavioral medicine faculty of the University of North Texas, has traveled throughout Mexico, seeking out native healers and attempting to objectify their healing testimonies. He reports that they appear to be successful with "preclinical" syndromes usually related to stress and anxiety factors. He also indicates that some patients of healers demonstrated physical changes attributable directly to the healers' methods.

Knowing how curious I am, many healers have requested to demonstrate their art in my clinics. I selected one of these individuals, Carolyn, to interact with some pain patients for two days in order to study what results her practice might bring about in their suffering, what we might learn from her successes, and how the patients would relate to her in the hospital environment. The patients were impressed with her abilities to intuit their past histories, and at least two of them experienced remarkable reductions in their pain and stress levels. In the most dramatic example, one of the patients reported that he had felt the presence of God in Carolyn and that he was cured by this remarkable woman. In another, less dramatic, incident, the patient attributed numerous improvements in his condition to this healer.

The patients were respectful of Carolyn and her talents and found it easy to talk with her. They all thanked me for bringing her to the clinic even if they experienced no healing personally. When I asked Carolyn what she did to accomplish the healing, she gave me a general explanation. She said that she became a conduit for God, allowing His energies to flow through her in the form of love. When I asked if anyone, such as myself, could heal in this manner, she assured me that if I could allow my mind to release its rational process and focus upon the patient with pure love, healing could take place. After Carolyn left, I began to attempt this process of healing as instructed. I soon learned that having a critical mind does not help; I had to open up beyond it. Then, to some degree, patients began to respond to my efforts. Though I do not consider myself a "healer," in some cases I found that if I could maintain an altered state of consciousness with full focus on the patient, I could seemingly effect documented changes in pain symptoms in the patient. I began to teach patient groups these approaches, using the community spirit as an additional component, and the technique appeared to yield impressive results. Because of the multidisciplinary team approaches employed in the clinic, physical changes attributable to the "healings" would have been very difficult to determine. For reasons discussed later in this chapter, I found it problematic to articulate a general program with this component as part of an allopathic medical protocol, nor did I deem it important to create one. I felt that the process itself (sending love and caring to healees) was inherent in all therapies. However, it did become a part of the group meetings for the patients.

One patient had been in a shipping accident about a year before admission into the clinic. The vertebrae in his thoracic region had been crushed by a crane, causing tremendous pain. After a staff member focused upon him using Carolyn's technique, his pain abated. As in the other case studies, I did not have new radiology tests run in order to prove a point; however, based on his subjective level of pain and his behavior, we know that there was a significant change.

What seemed remarkable about these cases was how well they demonstrate the underlying principles of the healing process. The basic assumption was that selfless, altruistic imagery would have some effect on another's being. Whether the imaging was in the form of a prayer or a focus of love, the primary goal was to maintain a clear regard for the healee without becoming involved with the outcome as a power issue. The major goal was to enhance the patients' well-being rather than taking credit for healing them. The potential for the development of the ego trip of "being a healer" was problematic for many reasons, discussed later.

I found myself conducting quasi-experiments, attempting to determine the reality of the apparently overriding connection between the imagery and the well-being of the patient, so profoundly demonstrated in some cases. It was uncomfortable for me to assume an energy field that encompassed all consciousness, unmeasurable with existing technology, even if it served in powerful ways. More frustrating was the ethical issue of the attitude of the health care provider if it seemed to create a positive or negative effect on the outcome of the case. For example, if a patient did not respond positively to a procedure, could the physician's attitude toward the patient be a factor? There were some staff therapists whose negative attitudes toward the biofeedback equipment appeared profoundly influential. When these individuals attempted to administer biofeedback interventions, the equipment would consistently fail. Modules would lose their electricity immediately in their hands, yet would revive their capacities once they were turned over to another person. Needless to say, the staff personnel who had the negative experiences with the machines consistently held the equipment in contempt and fear. The question remains: Is there an interaction of consciousness between individuals that cannot be explained by psychological or behavioral cues of stimulation?

Scientific Documentation
of Transpersonal Imagery

Very few studies have been conducted that would prove conclusively
the reality of a transpersonal relationship of consciousness; however,
there are many that might support an existing belief in the phenomenon. Much of the early work on experimentation on the relationship
of consciousness between organisms began in Russia. Ivan Pavlov considered clairvoyance a special facet of human consciousness; Vladimir
Bekhterev conducted laboratory experiments of telepathic influence in
dogs and in remote hypnotic influence of humans in his Institute for
Brain Research at the University of Leningrad in 1922.[5] Much of the
distant mental suggestion work was carried out by Leonid Vasiliev,
who developed technology and supportive evidence for a "second sig-
naling system" as an extension of the conditioning model of learning.
Vasiliev's work was published in English in 1976, under the title of
Experiments in Distant Influence, in which he details the methods that
he and his co-workers used to study distant influence (mental suggestion) on selected subjects.[6] Apparently it was from these interests that
the original technology for the EEG was developed.

In a series of carefully controlled experiments, Vasiliev used highly
selected subjects having great suggestibility at a variety of distances (20
to 1,700 kilometers) from the influencer. The general findings were
that there were demonstrable results, even through iron-, lead-, and
Faraday-chamber screening. The results of these pioneering efforts indicate that with distant suggestions (imagery), individuals can induce
motor acts, project visual images and sensations, influence sleeping/
awakening events and physiological reactions (breathing changes, electrodermal activity of the skin).

William Braud has conducted the controlled studies most accepted
by scientists, running experiments in this field for more than thirteen
years with remarkable integrity. His general design is very similar from
one study to the next, allowing comparisons between any two sets of
results. The work is intended to measure the effects of distant influencing by individuals on a variety of biological systems of other people.
The experimental design ensures that none of the nonexperimental or

environmental influences can account for the results, guarding against subtle cues, recording errors, expectancy and suggestion effects (the placebo principle), artificial reactions to external stimuli, confounding internal rhythms, and chance correspondences.[7]

In a series of fifteen experiments, a subject sat in a comfortable room while his or her spontaneous skin resistance responses (SRRs) were monitored continuously by means of electronic equipment interfaced with a microcomputer. Skin resistance is a measure of how fast electricity can travel across the skin. The production of sweat reflects the degree of activation of the subject's sympathetic nervous system and, hence, the subject's degree of emotional, cognitive, and physical activation or arousal. Higher SRR activity is associated with physiological activation, whereas lower SRR activity reflects relaxation. These measures have been used with "lie detector" scans and biofeedback protocols for stress management. In a distant, separate room (twenty meters away), the experimenter was stationed with another person, the "influencer." The ongoing SRR activity of the distant subject was displayed to the influencer by means of a polygraph. As instructed, the influencer watched the polygraph as he or she attempted to exert a remote conscious influence upon the distant subject; hence, the influencer did have a feedback system to determine what effect he or she might have been having and could alter the approaches—imagery, focusing, or whatever other techniques appeared to be effective—accordingly.

Braud and his associates have conducted 323 sessions with 271 different subjects, 62 influencers, and 4 experimenters. Six of the fifteen studies yielded statistically significant results in the expected direction; 57 percent of the individual sessions were successful in showing that a person could influence the physiology of another individual from a distance. When the series as a whole was analyzed using a technique for combining scores, the statistical probability by chance alone of one person's remote influence over another person's physical state could have been only 0.000023. The cumulative effect size was 0.23 (meaning that 23 percent of the variance in the way the results came out could be explained by the experimental impact), which means that the impact of an influencer is certainly not robust in the experimental laboratory, but even such a small documentable cumulative effect could be a basis for the conclusion that there is some substance to the global "one mind" theory.

Braud and his associates also examined another aspect of global consciousness in "staring" experimentation. The laboratory arrangement for controlling all sources of external affect was very creative. The subject (termed the "staree") was attached to the SRR recorder in a comfortable chair, as in the "influencer" studies. A video camera was aimed at the subject approximately 45 degrees left of center from the staree's point of view. The person designated to focus attention on the subject—the "starer"—was instructed, according to the research method, to stare at the subject's image in a television monitor for a specified period of time.

The starer was given no feedback as to the response of the subject's SRR or any other information about the staree. In four separate efforts, the researchers found evidence that the staree's autonomic responses could discriminate whether or not the person was being stared at from a remote situation via television. They also found that some subjects were more sensitive to the impact of being stared at and that their performances could be predicted by their introversion scores on a psychological test, the Myers Briggs Type Indicator (MBTI).

What Braud and his associates have maintained and demonstrated through replicated and accepted methodologies is that consciousness does bridge between two or more individuals in yet undetectable pathways. The process may be learnable, and individual differences in sensitivities may influence it; but as far as research technology can measure this subtle phenomenon, a statistical probability exists that transpersonal imagery has a distinct impact.

Very dramatic results in this field have been claimed by the Maharishi Mahesh Yogi group; however, the studies are based solely on an in-house review. (I am always concerned about the use of propaganda in such organizations, and mine is not the only voice questioning their intent or objectivity.) Nevertheless, the results provide an interesting support for transpersonal imagery. Their general philosophy is that the effects of Transcendental Meditation (TM) practice by a few participants will have a generalized effect upon the immediate environment.

In terms of the theory of consciousness used earlier in this chapter, their belief is that if a small portion of the "great mind" can be calmed, then the other parts will also experience a calming response.

One study compared the crime rate in twenty-four American cities with populations of 10,000 to 100,000 in which more than one percent of the population were trained and practicing TM meditators (experimental group) with another matched twenty-four American cities with less than one percent practicing meditators (control group).[8] While the crime rate increased in the control cities, it significantly decreased in the cities in which people were meditating. The researchers claim that a group of 300 TM meditators who spent June 12 to September 12, 1978, in Rhode Island influenced the total crime rate, mortality (except traffic fatalities), auto accident rate, pollution, unemployment rate, and beer and cigarette consumption rates by meditating. The state of Delaware was used as a control state.

The book *The Maharishi Effect*, another in-house effort, summarizes thirty-eight projects conducted by TM researchers between 1974 and 1990, claiming that if 0.5 percent of the population is practicing TM, the following parameters will be affected.[9]

crime rate	hospital admissions
homicide rate	pollution
suicide rate	economic indicators
war deaths	cigarette consumption
infant mortality rate	beer consumption rate
automobile accidents	divorce rate
fire accidents	degrees conferred
air traffic accidents	patent application rate
rate of infections	worker strikes

Perhaps related to the research into the existence of guidance beyond time and space as we know them is the "psi" phenomenon in animals. Remarkable documentation exists of animals—mostly dogs, cats, and birds—who have been lost thousands of miles from home and have found their way to their families. One story tells of a dog who was left on a highway while the family was moving to a new location.

Weeks later the pet showed up at the new house, guided through strange landscapes and pathways by some mysterious orientation.

Transpersonal Imagery in Clinical Settings

Clinical studies that have used the principles of transpersonal imagery are difficult to isolate as pure examples of the application because it is hard to ascertain overlap with other psychological processes known to effect change in physical conditions, such as the placebo effect. One interesting research effort was published by Braud in which he demonstrated that individuals could influence from a distance the rate of hemolysis of human red blood cells.[10] Although the blood itself was not to be used in any medical context, the study provides some validity for a possible healing prototype in a relevant setting.

If red blood cells are maintained in fluids with a salinity similar to that of human plasma, the cells survive for long periods. However, if placed in a fluid having a salinity lower than that of plasma (such as distilled water or a very diluted saline solution), the corpuscles swell as the water moves through their semipermeable membranes. Eventually they rupture and release their hemoglobin content. The process of release creates an opportunity to measure the rate of decomposition accurately through a spectrophotometer (a clinical analysis using color bands to denote chemicals and life energy levels). In this way, one is able to observe the deaths of the blood cells in a very precise manner, determining the power of transpersonal imagery on the very essence of life at the cellular level.

In Braud's experiment, thirty-two subjects attempted to prolong the lives of red blood cells—using imagery and intent—in ten test tubes submitted to osmotic stress (diluted saline solution). Test tubes of red blood cells in identical solution were used as controls. In those blood samples on which the persons focused their intentions, the blood cells lived longer than the blood samples that received no caring focus. Overall, the matter of who the blood originally came from did not significantly influence the outcome, although there was a definite trend toward influencing one's own blood more powerfully than another's, which, with greater numbers in the study, may have been significant.

In a more specific medical issue, one researcher conducted what he called a "triple-blind" study of the effects of intercessory prayer-at-a-distance on children with leukemia.[11] Neither the people being prayed for, the people doing the praying, nor the treating physicians even knew that an experiment was in progress. Each month the parents and the treating physicians independently filled out a questionnaire asking whether the illness, the child's adjustment, and the family's adjustments were better, the same, or worse. Ten of the children were prayed for daily over a period of fifteen months, while eight children were in the control group. At the end of the fifteen-month period, seven of the prayed-for children were alive, compared with only two in the control group. The study was flawed in many ways: for example, there were no means of matching the children in the groups or their families, or of isolating other sources of transpersonal intervention.

In another oft-cited study, prayer was used to explain the differences in outcome of coronary patients.[12] In a group of 393 patients diagnosed with heart disease, two subgroups were matched as to age, severity of disease, and diagnosis. One of the subgroups was designated as the prayed-for group, and each patient—identified by name and diagnosis—assigned to prayer groups of three to seven "born again" Christians. The researchers evaluated only medically relevant variables—such as complications and infections—as well as a general severity scale (a scale measuring the severity and impact of a disease). Although the two subgroups were amazingly similar at the beginning of the study, at the conclusion of the study, the prayed-for group enjoyed a better health outcome across all measures. This study was also flawed in many ways: for instance, there was no way to know whether or not the patients in the control group had received transpersonal imagery intervention, such as prayer, from some other source. I also have other reservations about this study, relating to the data itself and the objectivity of the evaluation.

There are plenty of personal testimonies of healing that relate to the validity of transpersonal imagery and intent. There are also serious reports of "voodoo" and "hex" incidents that may be used as evidence of negative transpersonal influence. Although no studies have been published of situations in which a negative goal or intent has been purposely planned, the possible influence of such forces can be found in many anthropological reports.

PRACTICAL CONSIDERATIONS OF TRANSPERSONAL IMAGERY

Whether or not there is proof that some energy force or transpersonal influence exists between people, most people want to believe that one does. Consider the behavior of fans at a sporting event, for example. Everyone feels that he or she is part of the action, taking responsibility for events as the favorite team takes on the challengers, even to the extent of taking personally the resulting victory or loss. Perhaps this transpersonal imagery model helps explain the "hometown advantage" recognized by all sports predictors. This phenomenon cannot be explained by familiarity with the field or personal recognition, but all coaches acknowledge the power of community support.

Although some individuals apparently possess greater transpersonal influence than others, the effect is subtle in any case. If we look at studies of the "hometown advantage" phenomenon, we see that being the home team increases the chances of winning statistically by 0.30 or less, which translates into less than a 10 percent greater impact than chance.[13] A 10 percent greater chance of winning, or of predicting a win based on your team's being at home, is not a very powerful element unless all other factors are balanced. For example, if two teams are equal in all other ways, the impact of transpersonal infleunce via community support would make a significant difference.

In terms of disease and health, the awareness of the effect of transpersonal influence (such as love and a caring attitude) may be recognized by a health care provider. Certainly the attitude of the therapist should be consistent with the desired impact of the therapy. Furthermore, if the clinical situation is appropriate, it does no harm to organize a transpersonal protocol to enhance the result of the treatment.

As I indicated earlier in the chapter, I have structured treatment protocols using transpersonal principles. I will admit that the outcome of these programs may be more related to the role of community and group support than what would be statistically attributable to transpersonal imagery. We know that group support accounts for the majority of successes in nearly any type of rehabilitation program. However, this process of group support and transpersonal imagery is no different from the ones used by the shamans in their efforts to help their community members.

The steps that we used in the clinic's programs are taken from cross-cultural literature regarding the enactment of positive transpersonal influence. They are as follows:

1. One begins the process by reaching a deep state of calm, an altered state of consciousness.
2. One focuses with a pure sense of love on the individual who is to receive help and support.
3. As one's focus on the individual intensifies, one projects a caring energy toward him or her. In doing this, one might visualize projecting love from the heart or opening one's own soul to allow the love of God to come through. The implied request is to bring nurturance toward the person from whatever source—a god or goddess, the universe, nature, or an animal spirit—the caregiver believes in. It is a request, not a demand addressed to God or the universe, to help in some way. If a group is conducting the program, everyone might do this at the same time.
4. If a group is involved, the process can be enhanced by singing, dancing, humming, holding hands or touching, and/or breathing together.

The process of transpersonal influence is very well articulated in Virginia Hind's book *The Pebble People*. Virginia's husband, Aldie, was critically ill with cancer. Virginia asked each friend and family member to think about him at a particular time of day, to focus on his health and send healing thoughts and love. As part of the process, each person was also asked to send a pebble to him every time he or she prayed for him. The accumulation of pebbles became a symbol of love energy, as well as of the broad community that was supporting Aldie. Aldie rallied against the disease for some time while this transpersonal practice was continuing. His story illustrates the power of deep love and relationship through the ordeal of disease.

THE ETHICS OF TRANSPERSONAL IMAGERY

I am thankful that transpersonal imagery has only subtle influence. Otherwise, I might have fulfilled my mother's imagery of me as a physician specializing in internal medicine—specifically in her internal medicine—and I would be married to the tallest girl in town. (She always felt sorry for tall girls, because it was harder for them to get a date.) Needless to say, I would also be living close to her, and I would be the president of the choir in her church. It is probably a good thing that the transpersonal force is not as strong as our own free will.

The matter of free will is one of three important ethical concerns to be considered when dealing with other people's lives. As a health care provider, one might consider good health as the most important value in people's lives, yet often other things are more important, even to someone facing death or disability. One can never know the "contract" each of us has with the universe or our own spiritual paths. Each person assigns to his life its own special purpose, and these purposes differ widely. To feel that one knows what would be the best direction for another person's life can be presumptuous as well as illusionary.

The second issue concerns what I call "ego-tripping." I always have an uncomfortable feeling when someone introduces him- or herself as a "healer." It may be a true designation, especially in cases in which the person has produced a therapy or medicine that can reverse the process of disease. Or perhaps that individual has experienced the power of transpersonal imagery in working with others. However, to call oneself a healer implies that one is solely responsible for what must be seen as a two-way, not a one-way, process. It must be acknowledged that the person who is healed has as much to do with his or her own healing as a so-called "healer." Even Jesus Christ, our principle example of transpersonal influence, usually asked questions about the healee's faith or used the healing process as a lesson in order to make a point about the person's life.

When I was involved in the experience of trying to heal others through transpersonal influence, I found myself overly attached to the other person's progress. This is a good example of an ego trip, or perhaps an "ego trap." If the person did not respond as I had hoped, I felt disappointed and often angry. At times I would blame the patient for having no faith; I also felt paranoid about how other health care professionals would regard my work. Often the patients would lie about their condition, hoping to bolster my confidence and hopes. For example, once when I was experimenting with healing through hypnotherapy, I was trying to demonstrate how a patient would feel no pain when I stuck him with a pin. The demonstration went well, as the patient did not appear to notice being stuck. The class was impressed. But after class, when I was discussing the hynosis with the individual to see if there were any lingering suggestions, I reminded him of the pin demonstration. He said, "Boy! That hurt!"

Surprised at his response, I questioned him further, to which he responded, "I just didn't want to make you look bad. I thought you were doing a good job, and if I had expressed pain, it would have ruined the demonstration. Besides, I really *do* believe in this stuff."

The third ethical issue concerns another component of investing one's ego in the transpersonal process. Just as the "healer" may be tempted to take full credit for results, so the "healee" may be tempted *not* to take responsibility for helping to improve his or her condition. For example, I used to spend a great deal of time and energy using massage and hypnosis on patients who thereby often registered a significant improvement in pain levels but then seemed to become dependent on me and the treatments. As long as I was around to give a treatment, the patients would not change their lifestyles or attitudes. This pattern was especially characteristic of the low-back-pain and hypertensive patients. Even though I would suggest they practice relaxing, pacing their lives, and changing their environmental response patterns, nothing would change. In a few days they would be back to see me with the same symptoms as before.

As I imagined a future spent treating hundreds of returning patients, I considered the problems associated with the one-way model of healing. I concluded that over the long run it may be more destructive than constructive to use a healing procedure that doesn't accommodate patient responsibility. If the treatment doesn't allow the patient to take some responsibility for him- or herself, the patient can't take the opportunity that disease often offers to learn from its symptoms. Without some integrated effort to incorporate the "lesson" of the disease, the patient will find the disease returning. As long as there is an external agent to help, there is no motivation to change our lives or correct our paths ourselves. This is like the chronic cougher who runs from doctor to doctor for help, rather than quit smoking.

I have been privileged to work with people who, because of pain and/or disease, are undergoing major changes in their lives. In some cases even the most difficult and rare diseases have been "cured" or put into "remission." In virtually every such case, the individual takes full credit for the reversal of the problem, which I think is fitting. Witnessing these cases has enabled me to define healing in a new way—as the individual's awareness of and power to use methods and attitudes that engender harmony. Cessation of symptoms after external intervention without the partnership of the patient is not healing. In my experience, a symptom that disappears without the patient's addressing the dynamic behind it is likely to reemerge later, in the same or a completely different form.

There is a double edge to transpersonal imagery, often referred to as "voodoo." Victims of voodoo have been known to die from exposure to the destructive influence of an individual's or group's negative imaging efforts. Yet well-meaning family and friends can also negatively influence a patient's condition through their inherent belief system. For example, statements such as, "He is going to die anyway. I had an aunt who had what he had," or, "She will always have a bad back—we inherited it," can adversely affect the recovery of the patient.

CONCLUSION

If we can assume that transpersonal imagery has some influence on healing, then medicine, as a science and art, should recognize its effects in the methodology of research design as well as the application of therapeutic intervention. As we have seen, the power of transpersonal imagery is limited, and the impact may not be heroic. However, if life and death are held in a delicate balance, wouldn't it be unethical *not* to pray for the patient as standard medical protocol? If we knew that cancer patients live twice as long if they have a support group that prays for them, wouldn't it make sense for the medical team to consider such programs as they might consider a drug under the same conditions? In his book *Healing Words*, Larry Dossey makes an inspiring case for the value of prayer and transpersonal imagery, concluding that if we applied the same research efforts to the consistent reports of life extension through these methods that we do for drugs and surgery, these practices would be in every hospital in the country.

Transpersonal imagery is controversial because our understanding of it is not aligned to our current scientific models. Yet its practice and efficacy are increasingly recognized, and through many avenues—sports, business, and health. We are not very good at practicing it, because we receive little feedback from doing so; moreover, those of us in the medical field may be embarrassed to discuss it in scientific circles. However, it is time to acknowledge these tools. Doing so will spur us to further research their practicality and effectiveness and to utilize their impact for the benefit of each other and the community at large.

||≡|||

Interview with Larry Dossey, M.D.

Author of *Space, Time, and Medicine*, *Beyond Illness*,
Recovering the Soul, and *Meaning and Medicine*

Frank Lawlis: You have begun to define medical paradigms as Eras I, II, and III. Could you elaborate on these definitions?

Larry Dossey: I use Eras I, II, and III as shorthand to describe the healing methods used in the world today and to understand them in the context of history. The scientific approach that began to be applied in medicine around the 1860s is a fairly mechanistic approach and would be defined as Era I medicine. Examples of Era I medicine would be the use of drugs and surgery. What I call Era II medicine was called psychosomatic medicine fifty years ago but is now referred to as "mind-body medicine." It is any intervention that involves using one's own consciousness to affect one's own body. Examples of Era II medicine include biofeedback, imagery, prayer, and positive thinking. Era III medicine is fundamentally different: it is by nature nonlocal and transpersonal. It is not lodged in space and time, such as Eras I and II are. It rests upon the possibility that the individual mind can reach out through time and space and affect distant bodies. There is much evidence to support this possibility.

Although the effects of transpersonal imagery are not very strong in the laboratory, they are, nevertheless, there and cannot be ascribed to chance. Transpersonal imagery, prayer, and other nonlocal methods of healing are demonstrable and reasonable. There is a dark side to these methods as well that we are going to have to deal with if we incorporate Era III medicine into our general approach to healing.

FL: If the Western medical system were to adopt this Era III paradigm, how would medicine be changed?

LD: I think that the definition of disease would be changed in several ways. Currently, disease is conceived as a response to malfunctions that occur solely within the context of the individual. We say that they originate there, although the bacteria and virus may come from external sources. These can be explained by a Newtonian model of cause and effect. If the Era III approach were accepted, we would regard the causality factors of disease and health to rest not solely in one person, but throughout the community. We would look at it from the perspective of a global mind network, which would enlarge the concept of health and illness infinitely.

FL: It reminds me of the ancient practice of the shaman, who would bring the whole community into the healing process.

LD: These are parallel concepts. I think that the indigenous understanding of these principles is right on target, enlarging the context to include the community and the planet, Mother Earth. If Mother Earth is sick, then we are sick.

FL: Do you consider diseases like cancer and heart disease related to community or global consciousness?

LD: It is fascinating to consider illness, especially contemporary illnesses, such as AIDS, in this light. Most people would agree that the earth is being stressed to its maximum, and us along with it. Human beings are the greatest of all threats to the environment. Since the earth is a conscious and living entity, it may be its goal as a living organism to eliminate the threat to its life. So human beings, as the greatest threat, are being brought under control in their most productive years via disease. This would be an ideal way for Mother Earth to protect herself. Of course, this is purely speculation, but it may be relevant to a discussion of consciousness and intelligence in an unlimited context.

FL: Could AIDS be created by such a consciousness?

LD: If a particular disease would protect Gaia, AIDS would certainly serve that purpose better than any I know. It is a chilling idea, but something I would not discount.

FL: Could you comment about what you described as the "shadow side"?

LD: Most people prefer to think that the transpersonal process is "nice" or does not work at all. If you go to a laboratory, you will find a broad set of experiments showing that human beings can retard bacteria growth; they can inhibit the growth rate of fungi and seeds at a distance. Many of these organisms have an identical growth process to ours. If people can weaken a simple organism, the same process could extend to other, more complex, living creatures.

Also, there is an aspect to these experiments, done at Princeton Engineering Anomalies Lab under Robert Jahn, which shows that not only can human beings skew the outcome of random generators in computers, they can turn it in negative directions as well.

If we consider the anthropological research, the evidence for the dark side effects is better recognized. For example, in Hawaii there was a widely practiced tradition before the Christians came called the "death prayer." The shamans would pray someone on a distant island to death. The key point is that the process was totally nonlocal, without the victim knowing what was happening. This is documented by Max Freedom Long, who went to Hawaii in the early 1900s. He found that the victims all died in the same way. They would develop an ascending paralysis in which first the feet and toes would become numb and immobile. This feeling would climb up the body until it reached the diaphragm, when the person would die of suffocation. There is an identical disease today called the Guillain-Barré Syndrome. The cause is unknown. Perhaps in some of these diseases for which we have found no known cause, negative transpersonal factors should be considered. Some people may say that this is nuts, but I think we have to consider such a possibility. Unless we widen our ideas about disease, medicine will never understand it fully or progress in its treatment. I also wonder about some of the so-called psychosomatic illnesses. In some individuals with these types of illnesses, the psychological patterns simply do not apply and the prescribed treatments do not help. Emotionally healthy individuals suffer from back pain, irritable bowel syndromes, and headaches the same as anyone else. I would raise the question as to whether some nonlocal negative influences might be at work. I think that something like "psychic pollution" may have some influence in these diseases, but we simply have no idea what is going on.

FL: Does this raise a question about the existence of evil forces?

LD: I think that it does. That question is one I have danced around for a long time. It is part of the spiritual perspective in most other cultures. It may be necessary for a little evil to be in the world. Without it we might not recognize the good. You can carry this to health and illness. If we did not have illness, we would not recognize health.

FL: Do you believe in the concepts of consciousness and communication as articulated in the "hundredth monkey" story?

LD: I thought these concepts were valid until I learned that the story is only a metaphor. My personal opinion is that a small number of people with the same consciousness can have an effect upon a larger group. But that is my belief and faith, and I have no major research to support it.

FL: Would the concept of Era III medicine explain the *psi* phenomenon of lost animals?

LD: I think that it would be arrogant to believe that this consciousness is bound to humans. In fact, animals may be more sensitive to energy loops of consciousness because they do not have to wrestle with egos so much. Animals are solidly in the nonlocal loops.

IIII 4 IIII

RESONANCE

The Transpersonal Moment

O NE OF THE BASIC assumptions of transpersonal medicine is that some kind of energy that facilitates movement toward wholeness can be transferred among individuals. This energy is the primary component of the healing ritual, a process whose purpose is to "make whole." Hence, the underlying principle of interpersonal ritual is to heal the broken connection between the person and his or her universe. One of the experiences of healing is the recovery or rediscovery of the state of true union with another person, with family, the community, the world, and the universe.

Among individuals who have experienced a cure, a common description of what they feel is "blending into the cosmos" or becoming "one" with the Creator. Interestingly, healers and therapists themselves report having the same feeling when some major transformational process occurs: feeling at one with the patient, sensing a connection with the other person at their very roots, plugging into common imagery. A healing ritual is healing for both the healer and the healee, a joint pilgrimage toward wholeness.

If this sense of complete unity with another is so critical in healing, it would appear that the field of clinical psychology would train its students in the healing ritual. My training in clinical psychology was excellent. My graduate work was approved by the American Psychological Association, as was my internship. I spent two years researching the central ingredients of effective psychotherapy skills and another three years in private practice before achieving diplomate status from the American Board of Professional Psychology, Inc. I have been honored to receive fellow status with the Division of Clinical Psychology from the American Psychological Association for "scientific contributions to the field." I mention all of this to indicate what pride and enthusiasm I have had for the discipline of applied psychology. However, nothing in my training prepared me for the power of what I call the "transpersonal moment" in my experience as a therapist.

Being mindful of the rigid ethical rules and practical issues of the field, I had been successful as a psychotherapist. However, one day while I was working with a woman who was dealing with a skin disease, I experienced a deep caring feeling, a sense of being with her without the need to be her therapist, a professional, or even a friend. I felt the boundaries between us dissolve. I was aware of a deep conscious regard for her as a person and respect for her needs, yet the experience took me beyond any I had ever had with a patient before.

Although I reported nothing of my experience to the client, I did call upon a professional associate to process my unusual response to her. Together, we ruled out transference or countertransference, lust, or romantic love as underlying motivations for my feeling. And yet we were unable to pinpoint its source. Finally we decided that whatever it had been, at least I was aware of it. If it should prove to be a problem in the client's therapy, I would consider options later.

In our next session, the client explained how deeply she was touched by our previous session, and how useful it had been in helping her deal with some of her painful feelings about her past. She said that she had "felt" my presence as a genuine and caring support that allowed her to probe the areas she had not known existed before.

I was surprised and somewhat embarrassed at hearing about her breakthrough. I had said nothing, interpreted nothing, that would give my participation credit for her reactions. In our next few sessions, her progress was remarkable. I continued to hold her in my consciousness with the total regard I had experienced earlier; however, I did not discuss my process with her, nor did she bring any concern about our relationship into our remaining sessions. When she eventually terminated the therapy, our relationship was excellent.

The next time I was aware of such intense regard for another, I was working with a man who was dealing with his prognosed death. Again, I felt the merging of our consciousnesses combined with a feeling of openhearted caring for him, regardless of his decisions or his opinion of me as a therapist. Although I did not discuss my experience with him, he reported to me that he had felt a wonderful sense of "partnership" betweeen us; he had the imagery of our facing death together. We worked together only briefly because he was hospitalized and died the next week. However, interestingly enough I "felt" the exact time he died, although I was several miles away and did not know that he was dying at the time.

Although I cannot claim to have experienced these moments of deep conscious caring for all of the clients and patients with whom I have worked over the years, at those times that I have allowed myself to enter this particular state of consciousness, there has been a transformation, both for me and for the client. It is not a state into which I enter lightly; in fact, it has raised many issues for me in terms of my professional training, shaking my assumptions about myself as a clinical psychologist. For example, without another label for such an authentic caring response, I found myself putting these experiences within the context of sex or love. How could I "fall in love" with these clients, especially with so many of them? Was I embarking on an addiction to fantasy relationships within my practice of psychotherapy? If so—based on the excellent reports of success from the clients—was my state of mind helpful? I was confused by the fact that although the process was intensive and overpowering, my emotional response was not what I would call even affectionate, much less sexual. My concentration on the individual was deeper, at a core level, as if I were looking directly into the soul. The care extended to this soul was extended to my own as well. We were as one.

After many hours of self-reflection, reading, and searching, I concluded that what I experienced with these clients could best be described as "transpersonal moments of relationship." They do not arise from the pathology of unresolved conflicts of the unconscious. Rather, they are windows of cosmic realization that we, as humans, exist beyond our individual personalities. They are opportunities to discover the depth of our capacity to genuinely care for another individual. These moments involve a practice of surrendering to a higher level of being, and allowing the possible loss of the lower self. Those who have approached this dimension naively or somehow selfishly recoil at the first taste of dealing with repressed fear and true selflessness. Should we enter purposefully into this relationship with another person, it will transform us as well as the other.

Abraham Maslow described peak experiences as having no time or space boundaries.[1] The transpersonal moment is a relationship that is also suspended from those anchors of reality. In this quantum jump, we come to realize a new energy, a new capacity within us. This moment of revelation expands to all who are within it.

THE TRANSPERSONAL MOMENT AS SPIRITUAL RELATIONSHIP

In *I and Thou*, Martin Buber discusses how humankind could learn to relate to each other on a spiritual plane. He says that when we recognize relationship as sacred—I-Thou—the dimension of union takes on a broader spectrum of energy and respect. Buber notes, "I can neither experience nor describe the form which meets me, but only body it forth. And yet I behold it, splendid in the radiance of what confronts me, clearer than all the clearness of the world which is experienced. I do not behold it as a thing among the inner things nor as an image of my fancy, but as that which exists in the present. . . . And the relation in which I stand to it is real, for it affects me, as I affect it."[2]

In a similar vein, Matthew Fox says that only by seeing the spirituality in each other and assuming ourselves as sacred entities can we achieve a mutually caring society based on the awareness of our connections to each other as holy and divine. On the contrary, those of us in medicine and psychology are taught to be in relationship with others on an "I-it" plane, protecting ourselves from the perils of subjectivity and the possibilities of confusing roles and responsibilities.

I am reluctant to use the term *love* in this discussion, because the word has so many connotations. Yet none other expresses the intense caring quality of the transpersonal relationship. Richard Moss writes, "To embrace a love that is beyond the level of personal and sensual love is to enter an experience of such magnitude that the whole personal self is dissolved into it. At every point in my inner nature where I held to a memory or a need—the old ways of fulfilling myself—the greater energy turned this into pain. I was too small for the energy. I had to let go, to surrender, to grow. It wasn't until I reached harmony within the greater energy that I recognized this force was part of a larger reality. The feeling state of this recognition is a profound love, but its existence is not compatible with the rigid grip of ordinary awareness."[3]

In the middle 1970s, I was intensely interested in understanding relationships, and I was constantly testing out the structure of many models. As I had the luxury of working with graduate students who were more than eager to have topics for their theses, we explored every idea imaginable to define what dimensions initiated relationships and what dimensions were absent to the relationships that died. We examined relationships from psychotherapy to marriage to business to friendship. We found that most theoretical models had three dimensions; however, when we clustered descriptions of relationships by a statistical technique called factor analysis, we discovered that there were four.

First, there was usually a dimension of respect or dependency, meaning that one person was likely to depend upon another's wisdom and authoritative expertise in an area or circumstance. A second dimension that emerged we called "identification," meaning that people in the relationship had similar interests or goals. Problem-solving was the third dimension, indicating that the individuals' bond was based upon a mutual problem, foe, or threat.

The fourth dimension was one of caring, comforting, and supporting. For lack of a better name, we called it the "love/affection" dimension. It was this dimension that appeared to have the greatest predictive power for a variety of relationships: marital support for the rehabilitation of alcoholism, the success in juvenile delinquency rehabilitation, and the success in natural birthing, for example. What the data suggested is that if love and caring were present, regardless of the other resources, transformation was possible.

TRANSPERSONAL MOMENT AS RESONANCE

The most available metaphor for the transpersonal relationship in a psychotherapeutic setting was proposed by Virginia Larson, who called it "resonance."[4] After interviewing thirty-one experienced psychotherapists about this phenomenon, Larson pinpointed the following aspects of it:

1. Intense concentration on inner experience that spontaneously initiates an altered state of consciousness.
2. Therapist-client synchronization of even tiny movement patterns.
3. Therapist-client alignment to a similar frequency noted by palpable shift.
4. Momentary merging of therapist-client selfhood boundaries.
5. Therapists' immediate nonverbal understanding of the client's unacknowledged feelings.
6. Specific sensations and/or feelings somatically and/or kinesthetically perceived by the therapists.

Results of Larson's exploratory research indicated that resonance had beneficial effects for the therapist as well as the client. Its impact appeared to decrease the client's feelings of isolation and create safety and trust, so that difficult, painful, or frightening issues could be confronted. One of the summaries from the article captures the essence of the experience: "There was a moment of feeling separate yet being very connected. The energy changed as if there were an alchemy or movement into a strong vibration frequency which felt like a gift of meeting and understanding. Following this resonance experience, the therapeutic work progressed more quickly to deeper levels."[5]

The metaphor of energy harmony has been used frequently in the health and healing literature, partly because the concepts are parallel to all matter dynamics and partly because it is easy to understand the process at a fundamental level. Applying the metaphor to resonance has some interesting implications. The physics of reasonance can be seen in the behavior of atomic nuclei as they spin in characteristic frequencies and transfer energy in differing degrees. When there is equilibrium within a system, the field is considered to be at resonance when the average rate of energy transfer per cycle from an external agent is maximal. Furthermore, when two systems are vibrating together, there is an enlargement and augmentation of the patterns of both.

At the very essence of energetic infrastructure, the individual atom has its own system and harmonic organization. The orbits of the electron around the nucleus, or valence shells, are arranged according to the natural harmonic series. As a resonance with another system (another atom, another molecule) emerges, the overall potential for transmutation of the energy system is heightened.

As electroencephalogram (EEG) studies tell us, a level of consciousness can be shared by two or more people. Brain waves are organized according to the harmonic series (like auditory tones), where theta appears to be the fundamental tone, and alpha and beta are the second and third harmonics. If theta is 5 Hz (hertz, or cycles per second), to be in harmony, alpha rate would be 10 (twice the Hz). The results of one study on inducing synchronistic EEG in two individuals have clear implications for the resonance model.[6] This study shows that as two persons approach identical EEG levels of brain activity, their consciousnesses appear to tune in to each other. The subjects report similar images, emotions, and understandings of the world, even if they are not in close proximity to each other.

We have made similar observations when we use drumbeats to induce brain-wave stimulation. While a group of subjects listen to the same drum rhythms, similar symbols and images arise in the minds of several individuals at the same time. Sometimes deer will dominate the imagery, whereas bears might be the common image in the next experience. We have never attempted to program what images arise, and the possibilities of the group's having common images by coincidence is so small as to be nonexistent. Considering the new research[7] on the microtubes, the skeletal makeup of the nerves, and how one microtube vibrates at specific patterns, creating a communication among all other nerve cells, it makes sense that if a person "vibrates" at a specific frequency, that energy could be transmitted to others at some level. An understanding of this kind of communication would certainly bring a new perspective to our relationships.

Swaying together, standing and moving side to side and allowing ourselves to relax into the movement with our eyes closed, either with one other person or in a group, also results in mutual imagery and feelings. I have tried this with my patients. As we would move together, the transpersonal moment would occur, and boundaries of consciousness would fall away. I could direct the imagerial process as if I were on the journey with the client. The clients consistently reported a sense of total partnership in the experience. The perception is one of common flow of energy, as if we were going down a stream or river of energy in the same direction at the same speed, allowing us to tune in at the same precise level. It is no accident that these methods—along with dancing, singing, humming, and chanting—are used in shamanic rituals as a way to reach altered states of consciousness. Although the hypothesis has not been tested experimentally, I would expect that rhythmic physical movement induces brain-wave modification to theta patterns, as does the acoustical stimulation of drumming.

The metaphor of energy harmony is not only convenient but also appropriate to apply to the experience of transpersonal moments in relationship. As two individuals enter into an altered state of consciousness, allowing an opportunity for the consciousness to slow down, they enter into a mutual, commensurate energy state. A period of harmonic resonance develops and the sense of authentic sharing emerges. Since the energetic field is shared, the inherent separateness between the persons dissolves. The energy required to be a self, to maintain the "me," dissolves into a "we," and the imposed boundaries of selfhood merge, leading to a state of illumination.

Referring back to quantum physics, particularly in terms of "illumination," we could expand our metaphor. An unusually high number of patients who shift physiologically and psychologically express seeing a "light" in their imagery. The laws of quantum physics tell us that electrons that shift from one valence to another need energy. Shifting from the inner level to the outer level absorbs energy (catabolic), while shifting to an inner level gives off energy (anabolic).[8] Perhaps at an atomic level, this energy emitted in the form of light reaches consciousness in some associated imagery components.

IMPLICATIONS OF THE TRANSPERSONAL MOMENT

Many illnesses can be seen as disharmonies of the body and mind. For example, if we consider the immune system as a basic energy level, we can see how greater or lesser resonance with the inner or outer personal forces of the person can result in disease. If the immune system is hyperactive and out of resonance with other systems, the way it processes external factors—viruses, pollens, gases, and the like—will be categorized as a hyperallergic or ecological disorder. In the extreme, a person with such a disorder literally would be oversensitive to the world, which could result in death. If the imbalance is manifested internally, autoimmune disease will flourish. In such instances, the immune system is so sensitized and hyperreactive that it cannot tell the difference between self and nonself and will attack anything, including joints (arthritis), organs (lupus, diabetes), and nerves (multiple sclerosis).

As the table indicates, if the energy is hypoactive and does not react appropriately to the attack of other forces, disease will reveal itself.

IMBALANCE OF ENERGY LEVELS

	High Energy Systems	*Low Energy Systems*
Internal Imbalance	Autoimmune disorders	Cancer Immune deficiency
External imbalance	Hyperallergic reactions Ecological disease	Infection

Inability to protect itself against external threats—such as viruses or pollen—will result in infections. Inability to correct internal conditions, such as malformed cells and toxic invasions, will result in the development of such diseases as cancer and immune deficiency syndromes. Some of these imbalances can be traced to mental states, such as stress and depression; some can be traced to physical states such as biochemical imbalance or muscle confusion. However, sometimes the body and mind are simply so overwhelmed by external or internal activity that adaptation or skills are not available to develop appropriate responses. Obvious illustrations are traffic accidents and radiation exposure. Regardless of what force is acting upon the person, if the energy is not in proper resonance, disease is the natural outcome, a signal for change and transformation.

Dean Ornish has recently published the results of his pioneering study of an alternative approach to dealing with heart disease.[9] In this study he administered a program consisting of a major diet plan, a relaxation protocol, and moderate exercise and imagery to a group of people who had experienced a cardiac incident, while a matched control group was treated with traditional protocols. Most of the program was administered within the context of supportive group sessions. While earlier studies have noted that changed lifestyles such as diet and exercise could arrest the progress of cardiac disease, Ornish demonstrated that the disease could be *reversed*, a landmark finding.

The Ornish program contains many of the components found successful in other rehabilitation efforts; however, the primary significant factors that Ornish pinpoints differ from those in other programs and are also relevant to the transpersonal moment experience. He calls the pivotal process "the opening of the heart, the opening of the consciousness for love and caring to enter into the person's experiential frame of reference,"[10] the most important feature of the healing process. He credits the interpersonal influence of the community support as the critical factor.

Ornish's study has obvious implications for the importance of resonance and transformation. People who participated in the study experienced transpersonal bonding to a degree that they had never known before. Many of those who allowed themselves to be transformed by this experience consider their disease a blessing, the grace that transformed their lives and blended their souls with others' through resonance and caring.

The nonspecific syndrome called hyperallergic or clinical ecological disease has reached epidemic proportions. People suffering from this condition have increasing sensitivities to vague and subtle forces, often stemming from new food processing technologies and/or the materials from which our clothing and houses are made. My colleague Bob Butler and I, both of whom have worked as clinicians and researchers in this field of medicine, have come to the conclusion that our minds and bodies are taxed and confused in their attempts to adapt to the increasing complexities of environmental forces in which we are literally bathed. The immune system, our protective system, as well as our consciousness, becomes confounded in its own resonance. "Chronic Fatigue Syndrome" is often the long-term diagnosis.

The only approach that I have witnessed as being consistently helpful to these patients is to somehow recover resonance within their systems. Often this recovery can be achieved through imagery and biofeedback techniques. However, the most dramatic outcomes I have seen have been through the caring and loving presence of another person. It takes time and support, but healing back to harmony can and does happen.

In 1991 Dr. Benjamin L. Crue addressed the American Academy of Pain Management with one of the most compelling speeches I have ever heard on the treatment of chronic pain. Dr. Crue, who has directed a pain clinic for thirty-two years, is a pioneer in neurological surgery who has devised new techniques and procedures in the alleviation of suffering. His topic had to do with the controversy about the treatment of fibromyalgia, a severe pain disorder related to chronic muscle spasms that might occur anywhere in the body but is responsible for a great portion of back and neck pain. One school of treatment advocates a local treatment such as physical therapy and anesthetic blocks. The other school argues that since the pain symptom probably results from brain dysfunction akin to a local epileptic seizure in the motor area, treatment such as biofeedback, counseling, or biochemicals should be limited to that area.

During that keynote address Dr. Crue discussed his insights into the nature of chronic pain, especially focusing on our ignorance of the nature of pain and how to deal with it. He concluded that the best, and perhaps the only successful, treatment for this syndrome is "love." In this discussion he pointed out that the fibromyalgic patient's underlying energy level is in a cycle of ongoing crisis. At a neural level, the brain is constantly overcharging the body, namely the muscles, without a release signal. In a caring atmosphere and community, the energy can be transmuted and focused for a broader experience of self-acceptance and opportunities for peaceful self-love. In Dr. Crue's experience in treating pain, which is identical with my own clinical findings, those patients who can be exposed to the healing resonances of others, regardless of professional training or rank, have the greatest probability of healing.

The Transpersonal Moment in Transformation

People faced with the challenge of major disease can experience transformation to a degree that they probably never touched before. A confrontation with the possibility of death or long-term dependency brings us to honest terms with ourselves and those around us. It is said that "cancer cures neurosis," and in many cases, this is true. The patient feels an urgent need to prioritize his or her values, allowing what is of illusionary value to fall away. Many people think that what I do professionally must be depressing because it involves witnessing the deaths or decay of people I care about. Actually it is a wonderful experience to share what can be the most genuine moments of a person's life. If there is a period in someone's life when honesty comes to the fore and character comes clear, it is at this time. There is no longer any reason for pretense, denial, or speculation about future events such as becoming rich or poor, growing old, or spending time in jail. It is my privilege to be with these people, to share their emotional nakedness and their genuine presence.

At the same time, the friction of the pain and disease of terminally ill patients appears to create energy and the need for genuine relationship and love. Throughout our lives—especially if we are men—we are taught to defend ourselves from allowing people to see our inner motivations, our true intent, by "keeping our cards close to our chests." We learn to communicate so that only our most acceptable selves show. However, when time is running out, we often suddenly feel the isolation and loneliness of a lifetime from which a truly caring, open attitude has been absent. The onset of disease engenders further feelings of isolation, as we are suddenly seen as a "sick" person in the community. At the same time, communicating with others can become more difficult as our own major issues shift radically away from the mundane.

Higher energy states are required to transmute the reality of illness, which can seem unchangeable. Especially with the onset of anxiety and loss of self-esteem, there is a tendency for the increased flux of the patient's energy to weave a defensive net around the self, a self-protection against the onslaught of change. Patients strive to empower the old reality until they find the safety and direction of consciousness expansion and transcendence. Yet to a great degree our scientific medical world attempts to fortify the reality that may have itself produced the disease state. We answer or wave off the deep questions, sedate the anguish, and in every way possible try to lower the energy state, instead of joining and channeling it. For example, even though a patient's mental rehearsal of the healing process has been shown to be helpful in presurgical protocols for enhancing healing, his or her reduced emotional arousal may actually have a detrimental effect. Surprisingly, complications and delayed healing measures are correlated with the simple notion of calmness, be it chemical, social, or even religious. The underlying need is not to sedate, but to marshal and fine-tune the patient's resources in order to deepen the transformational process.

At one level or another, nearly every human being attempts to continue familiar life patterns until some force comes along to incite a new dynamic. There are people who have energy and money poured into their treatment by doctors and hospitals so that they can sustain their old lives because they are afraid or simply don't know that they can begin to harness the current of their being and direct it toward health.

All healing procedures—an injection of steroids or antibiotics, laying on of hands, surgery, counseling, acupuncture, chiropractic, or whatever—are essentially energy modification techniques. What I mean by this is that they tend to interact with each other, influencing the system to either stimulate or sedate the level of activity, either specifically or generally. Whatever the intended physical response, the goal of the spirit is not to return to the homeostatic being that existed before the onset of disease but to evolve to the next level of consciousness. Through the awakening levels of consciousness, not only do we experience the self as a dance of energetic interactions transcending our ideas and beliefs, but we also recognize that the process of living far transcends our relative goals. A strong and powerful sense of caring, a special kind of love, from another being can provide the grace and energy for transformation. By resonance with another person, transcendence to other realities and perspectives can be achieved. The wholehearted participation of all the individuals involved in caring for a patient results in our awareness of the infinite possibilities within each of us. The process can also reassure us that the mysteries of the universe are fundamentally altruistic.

As health care providers, we could take as our responsibility to enter into relationship with each other in order to establish an atmosphere of resonance. This would help bring about others' transformation as well as our own. To do so would require courage, honesty, and intent, qualities we do not teach in our medical schools or universities, yet among the most profound of all healing principles. Resonance brings about transformation for the individual human spirit, but it also brings a unity of all participating human spirits. Perhaps this is the best definition of healing love of the community. This principle of union is clearly demonstrated by the loving and forgiving ceremonies of the master ritualist as he or she organizes the process toward a common altered state of consciousness. However, in my opinion, this principle does not require demonstration for further proof. There is, however, an urgent need throughout the world—a need not for proof, but for demonstrated action of the principle itself.

A Cautionary Note

The transpersonal moment has natural healing potentials. There are no maps of how this interaction can be harnessed and propelled. Resonance is not simply loving another person, although that aspect certainly has some important dynamics. What is also necessary is for the healing professional to be willing and able to allow him- or herself to enter into the energy field of the patient and mobilize the spirit toward the evolution it deserves. There are many unknowns about the transpersonal moment: perhaps it can be directed, perhaps it stems from the unconscious—perhaps both. In any case, it is not a readily controllable phenomenon. For example, it is difficult for me to quickly muster up the intensity required to find this moment with another person. The process requires the development of sacred space, a safe relationship, and a mutual intention to explore the mysteries of other realities. Many therapists and spiritual leaders have said that this space is dangerous to the soul; they typically solicit power animals to accompany them on their journeys.

I should caution against the unbridled and enthusiastic use of resonance. This kind of deep work requires wisdom, maturity, experience, and skill. Without some level of maturity and knowledge of how to channel the energies that result, there is a danger of misguided or egotistical motivations. It is easy to confuse the emotions that the transpersonal moment evokes, for example. Also, a balanced and mature perspective is requisite. There are several stories of students and enthusiastic therapists who have experienced serious problems from being so deeply involved with another person. One of my students who was particularly sensitive became too absorbed in the energy fields of a dying client, losing her own boundaries and ability to let go of the process. I felt that the experience indirectly resulted in her own death from diabetes two months after the client died.

With the awareness of one's own vulnerability, one has the opportunity to enter into the resonance of another, to experience the transpersonal moment in relationship. Here I have tried to elucidate the dimensions of ambiguity and uncertainty; there are also the continuing distractions of unconscious fears. However, used properly, the transpersonal moment provides an inner path for transformation that has the power to reintegrate both healer and healee into the community as well as into a harmonious balance of body, mind, and spirit.

‖‖≣‖‖

Interview with Dean Ornish, M.D.

Author of *Dr. Dean Ornish's Program for Reversing Heart Disease*

Frank Lawlis: You have successfully demonstrated that human beings have the potential for reversing heart disease through participation in your program, which includes group support, diet, and exercise. What do you think is the primary factor for success in this approach?

Dean Ornish: I have used the image of "opening the heart" a great deal. Although at first, participants in the program see each other as very different in terms of socioeconomic status and personality, sharing only their heart disease, as we meet in support sessions people begin to trust one another and are able to express their feelings. So often they talk about how lonely and isolated they feel. The epidemic in America is not just physical heart disease but also spiritual and emotional heart disease. In this culture it is hard for us to realize that even though on one level we are separate from each other, on a deeper level we are all connected to each other.

Although these people are different from each other, they begin to discover the similarity of their feelings, especially their isolation and loneliness. They feel that such loneliness must mean that they are somehow lacking; otherwise they would not be feeling so bad. At some level everyone remembers what it feels like to be connected with someone else. "If only I had that something or ——, I would not feel so lonely anymore." We try to fill that space with different things— money, sex, power, whatever. All of these people felt this way, but once they had filled in that blank, they found that it really did not bring what they thought. They actually felt more stress. Rather than gaining respect and love for being a success, they often attracted envy. Success, or whatever, might bring some sort of love for a short period of time, but it does not last for long. Then we begin to search for something else.

Until we get "it," we feel stress; if someone else gets "it," we feel more stress. This reinforces the view of the world as a hostile, aggressive, zero-sum kind of place, and the stakes go up. One becomes a "winner or loser" who is on the line. Losers are more isolated than ever, and winners are respected. One patient said, "I could not enjoy being at the top of the mountain because I could see another one to climb. The letdown I felt after accomplishing one goal was so great that I had to have dozens of goals going on at the same time so I would not have to think about it."

There is a definite need for connection among people. I suppose that one of the reasons is that we do not have within our culture the usual ways of getting this need met anymore; we have few extended families, few nuclear families, few neighborhoods that we grow up in, no lifetime jobs, no long-lasting social institutions to give us a place where people feel connected, can feel who they really are.

That is not to say that we shouldn't have protective walls, but if there is always a wall between us and others, the same walls that protect us also isolate us. What we found is that if we could provide a safe place for people to begin opening their hearts to each other, then we could create a real community. And that became a very important reason for people to stay in this program—more important than their clogged arteries, blood pressures, or any other physical reasons that brought them to it.

The rewarding aspect of this work is that although people get into the program for basic survival reasons, what keeps them is that their lives improve in so many other more meaningful ways. We know that the ancient ways of healing were not for the purpose of unclogging arteries or lowering blood pressures—they are more powerful than that. They were for transformation and ultimately to transcend that isolation that is the root of so much illness. I have come to understand that stress comes not so much from what you do, but how you react to what you do.

To be able to work with ill persons in using their experience as a catalyst for transforming their lives, for opening their hearts in a non-physical sense, is an opportunity we do not take advantage of as professionals. There is a window of opportunity to channel our intentions at that time, and it is easy to miss it.

FL: In your work with some of your patients, I thought that the interpersonal dynamics were stressed. Do you perceive a changed state of relationship between the patients as healing begins to take place?

DO: Let's go back to the model we discussed before—"If only I had ——, then I would not be isolated"—which is a model of deprivation. What we strive to present to our patients is that meditation and community support are powerful techniques that can quiet the mind so that the person can begin to feel inner peace and well-being. Peace and well-being arise not because the person got what they needed or filled in the blank with the "right" thing, but because they are no longer disturbing what they already have. That is a real paradox. This new experience can reframe their worldview. Instead of seeing the world as unfair because we are not getting what we "need," we begin to ask: What am I doing to disturb the inner peace that I have in the first place? This engenders a sense of empowerment.

As people begin to open their hearts to each other and also to quiet their bodies and minds, an energy arises. They begin to look better; their skins take on a healthier tone; they feel better. That is what makes the difference. They can see each other begin to heal, and everyone takes joy in that. At the end of every session we ask everyone to hold hands. This allows us to *feel* the connection among all of us.

‖‖ II ‖‖

BEYOND
THE SELF IN
VERTICAL
SPACE

‖‖ 5 ‖‖

ALTERED STATES OF
CONSCIOUSNESS

W E HAVE SEEN THAT transpersonal medicine is aligned with the
search for wholeness and harmony beyond the rational self.
Basic to the process of moving into that space has been the need to
achieve an altered state of consciousness (ASC), a major pathway to
physical and psychological healing. In general terms, an ASC is a state
of reality that is separate from our normal, day-to-day reality. There
are many ways to achieve an ASC. In this chapter we will discuss the
methods that are most effective in the therapeutic setting; what dangers, if any, are involved; what psycho-neuro-physiological mechanisms lie behind an ASC; and what scientific evidence points to its
usefulness as a healing tool.

Soon after I became interested in healing, I was offered the opportunity to establish and direct pain clinics in major hospitals in Texas
and New Mexico. The mission of the pain clinics was to administer
"behavioral" techniques to those patients for whom conventional medical treatments had not been successful. Even though the clinics were
set up in locations that are among the most conservative in the United

States, I found that genuine concern on the part of the medical staff for their patients frequently motivated them to try techniques that had not been officially sanctioned by the medical establishment.

Since the patients at the clinics were by definition failures of conventional medical treatment, we knew that any successful treatment would have to be unconventional or extraordinary. If our methods were successful—measured by the comfort that the patients experienced—and if the programs attracted referrals from the medical community, our work would be accepted. Ultimately, the programs would be evaluated on the results we produced. It was with this license that ideas were constantly challenged, modified, accepted, or rejected; but we always examined them with the aim of understanding our explanations of success by investigating a wide variety of healing metaphors.

During the first two years of the clinic's operation in Texas, I personally experienced being in a sensory-deprivation "flotation tank," a large tub totally enclosed in darkness with approximately eighteen inches of salt-saturated water heated to ninety-five degrees. The experience impressed me. In the flotation tank, I became acutely aware of my body, especially of the tension of my muscles. I also reached a deep and profound sense of relaxation and peace. I immediately began to consider the benefits of this treatment for patients with severe muscular tension and chronic pain. After a review of the literature about the application of flotation devices (of which there was very little), I requested a trial for the clinics.

Installation of the tanks was fraught with problems from the start. There were concerns about maintaining hygiene and constant temperatures (salt crystallizes at temperatures close to ninety-two degrees and clogs up the filters), wax-dissolving properties of the salt solution (creating damage to floors when patients walked back to their rooms), and leakage. When I finally decided to abandon the idea, a hospital engineer volunteered to help design a workable apparatus. The final result was something of a combination between a sensory deprivation chamber and a water bed, but it did meet the specifications of the hospital. We were able to begin a serious trial period of monitoring the patients who underwent this particular therapy with biotechnological instrumentation such as the recordings of the electroencephalograph (EEG) and electromyograph (EMG).

As I had suspected, patients who used this device did become more relaxed. However, something even more important happened. Patients were being gently and safely introduced to what many of them referred to as "a different world where there was a total loss of personal boundaries and peace." One patient explained that she felt "God's love" while floating in the tank. Another patient described the sense that she understood "everything" from her experience in the chamber. We discovered that some of the patients would often slip into the chamber, sometimes at night, and spend long periods in the peacefulness and safety of the enclosure without our knowledge. Later it occurred to us that what they were doing was inducing an altered state of consciousness.

The staff and I became concerned that we might have instigated some form of psychotic behavior, and we were afraid that the patients' physical conditions would deteriorate. We were seriously considering disposing of the chamber. However, as it turned out, just the opposite proved to be true; the conditions of the patients significantly improved. Their reports of decreased pain and other symptoms were highly correlated to their use of the chamber. Moreover, the patients appeared to gain in psychological terms—there was less depression and more energy. What symptoms remained, such as pain or tissue damage, became almost a secondary concern to the patients as feelings such as love and peace emerged as primary issues.

As far as experiences with altered states of consciousness go, we observed similar results after prolonged exposures to drumbeats or other acoustical rhythmic stimulation, some selections of music, breathing exercises, and imagery therapy. However, with the flotation chamber, one important benefit was that patients could experience their altered state of consciousness for longer periods of time without needing a staff member to help them. The chamber was also more socially acceptable—they could show it to friends and relatives without a sense of embarrassment about "flaky, head-trip stuff," like drumbeats and imagery.

When patients were asked to describe what they experienced in the flotation chamber or through other various techniques for producing an ASC, there was a surprising consistency in their reports. All patients experienced the following feelings to some degree:

- A feeling of spiritual love (not attached to a specific person or thing)
- A connection to a universal community (being part of a plan greater than one's own)
- A deeper sense of self (autonomy, self-esteem, the belief that "I matter")
- A sense of goals beyond personal needs (altruism, compassion, humanitarian impulses)
- An understanding of problems (free from having to find a solution)
- An understanding of many levels at once (being able to see the same issue from many vantage points)
- A sense of being "real" yet with no boundaries (personal authenticity within a larger reality)
- A frustration at putting their experience into words (having witnessed a reality that words cannot describe)

In spite of the apparent wisdom they felt had been engendered through their altered states of consciousness, none of these patients were particularly more insightful in their counseling sessions. Their problems did not dissolve, nor were they more insightful into others' issues. However, they were less anxious about life questions, less depressed about not finding the answers. They continued to work hard in both physical and psychological therapies, and their motivation did not suffer. Our conclusion was that ASC changed their perspectives about their lives, but not necessarily in ways they could articulate.

What Is an Altered State of Consciousness (ASC)?

One scientist describes the state of altered consciousness as "any mental state(s) induced by various physiological, psychological, or pharmacological maneuvers or agents, which can be recognized subjectively by the individual himself (or by an objective observer of the individual) as representing a sufficient deviation in subjective or psychological functioning from certain norms for that individual during alert, waking consciousness."[1] Another defines it in biological terms as "a specific pattern of physiological and subjective responses—cortical, autonomic, and somatomotor functions on the one hand, simultaneously occurring imagery, ideation, and fantasies on the other."[2] However, a third scientist best describes the general perspective as a shift of focus, structure (one's awareness of oneself being aware), attributes of perceptions (images, thoughts, feelings, and memories), and disruptions or changes in the flow of thought. Included in this broad category would be daydreaming, meditation, hypnosis, and sleep dreaming.[3]

The following characteristics—adopted from the works of Arnold Ludwig, Arthur Deikman, and Charles Tart[4]—delineate how ASC differs from ordinary consciousness:

> Alterations in thinking
> Disturbed time sense
> Loss of control
> Change in emotional expression
> Body image change
> Perceptual distortions
> Change in meaning and significance of perceptions
> Sense of the ineffable
> Feelings of rejuvenation
> Hypersuggestibility
> More intense sense of reality
> Unity
> Altered feedback in consciousness network

It may be useful to distinguish the characteristics of altered states of consciousness from those of states that are noted as pathological (psychosis, dissociation, etc.). Although there may be some similarities with the categories listed, many of them do not apply to states of psychosis. For example, one who experiences a psychotic episode often describes it as "less real than ordinary reality," as opposed to more real. Within the psychotic experience, there is also often a "splitting of realities," which is definitely not a function of altered states of consciousness. Those individuals experiencing true ritual ASC express a sense of universal unity and connectedness, the opposite of schizophrenic thinking.

One group of researchers compared the experiences of altered states of consciousness among schizophrenia patients, individuals in hallucinogenic drug states, and people who had had mystical experiences. Through extensive multidimensional scaling techniques, they concluded that the descriptions of the experiences of each group were different enough that they could actually be used to accurately determine the group to which each person belonged.[5]

Altered states of consciousness are typically measured in terms of subjective experience and description; however, biological changes have also been used to measure shifts of consciousness. For example, decreased sympathetic arousal, increased parasympathetic activity, shifts away from ordinary cerebral activities (reduced control of the dominant, verbal-analytic hemisphere and asynchronous EEG activity), and increased hemispheric equivalence as indicated by greater hemispheric synchronization have all been shown to be symptomatic of altered states of consciousness.[6]

Although there has been much excitement about the potential for a biological definition of altered states of consciousness, no specific technological measurement can be designated to signify an "altered state." A few case studies using the new measurements of BEAM (Brain Electrical Activity Map) and imagery do tend to confirm the theoretical explanation of different brain symmetry differences.[7] The measurements consistent with the subjective descriptions of altered states have been of high magnitude within the *theta* range of function. In case the reader does not know the terminology of EEG ranges, there are only four basic categories:

beta: greater than 13 Hz (cycles per second)
alpha: 8 to 12. 5 Hz

theta: 4 to 7.5 Hz
delta: 0.5 to 3.5 Hz

Most of our mental activities in everyday life—problem-solving, worrying, planning—take place in the *beta* range. *Alpha* is the state we normally refer to as the relaxation state, when the mind is calm and restful. In this state, we can still monitor ordinary reality, and even train our brains to produce high alpha waves through the use of bio-feedback EEG technology. Theta range is that state between conscious and unconscious control, such as the drowsy state we feel just before going to sleep, when the boundaries between spheres of categories of perception merge. For example, if the telephone rings in an adjacent room we might or might not be able to tell if the ringing is real or in our dreams. This is the time of greatest creativity because it offers opportunities to mix realities and look for symbolic form.

According to reports by inventors, who must utilize both their technical knowledge and their imaginations, the theta state provides them with the greatest access to all levels of material. We know that many inventions and scientific discoveries—the sewing machine and the carbon ring, for example—were made while their innovators were in a theta state. Unfortunately, because the theta state happens in a withdrawal from ordinary reality, it cannot be trained with the use of self-monitoring devices.

Finally, the delta range is produced when we are in a sleep state without reference to conscious process. It is characteristic of deep dreaming sleep.

Melinda Maxfield conducted one of the best controlled research projects for the production of altered states by exposing her subjects to different patterns of shamanic drumming for thirty minutes at a time and comparing EEG ranges in a mixed intervention design.[8] Acoustical stimulation of a constant speed is thought to drive brain waves in predictable patterns, and with the definition of a shamanic pattern of four to seven beats per second (the same speed as the theta range), it was hypothesized that the brain patterns would react in accord with subjective experiences of an ASC. In all subjects, the altered state was confirmed by both the subjective experience and EEG readings.

This study has major implications for further research and clinical application of the altered state experience. The direct clinical approach for our patients was to administer acoustical stimulation (drum beats) and have them experience altered states within the short period of fifteen minutes, which is a far more efficient means of achieving a shift than being trained to achieve the same level of awareness through biofeedback or relaxation.

There are a number of stituations where we can observe, on a subjective basis, shifts from ordinary to nonordinary reality. Some of these methods can be itemized singly or in combination:

1. Sensory Deprivation
   Solitary confinement[9]
   Prolonged social deprivation[10]
   Extreme boredom[11]
   Total body-cast experience[12]
2. Overstimulation
   Brainwashing[13]
   "Mob trance"[14]
   Firewalkers trance[15]
   Shamanistic trances[16]
   Fugues, amnesias, traumatic neuroses resulting from severe
      emotional impact[17]
3. Relaxation and Trance Experiences
   Mystical or revelatory inductions[18]
4. Physical Deprivation[19]
   Hypoglycemia
   Dehydration
   Thyroid and adrenal gland dysfunction
   Sleep deprivation
   Hyperventilation
   Temporal lobe seizures

How Does ASC Work?

The evidence suggests that if guided and structured appropriately, altered states of consciousness can be of enormous benefit for most people, especially those in need of personal transformation. To know when an ASC is appropriate depends, in large part, on an understanding of its underlying mechanisms—not only how it works but on what parts of the human being it has its greatest impact.

ASC appears to work through a process of destructuring and re-structuring the mental and emotional framework of one's world. One researcher has worked out a "deautomatization" explanation of this sequence.[20] As individuals mature, there is a tendency to develop an automatization of responses, both mentally and physically. For example, when learning to ride a bicycle, one must first concentrate on both motor skills and perceptual judgment to keep the bicycle up and going in the right direction. As these processes are learned, they become habitual—automatized—and the learning process that led to the stage of completion is quickly forgotten.

Because of the automatization process, one remembers how to ride a bicycle and can respond quickly to different situations without thinking through the necessary reactions each time. However, associations with the process that may not have constructive attributes are also automatized, such as frustration in dealing with an angry parent or competition with a sibling. These associations are also forgotten and may be difficult to capture through memory.

An altered state of consciousness can provide the opportunity for deautomatization, the undoing of the habitual patterns. In this state we are able to revisit the experience and recall not only the events of the primary learning process but also the subjective issues associated with it. Since automatization normally accomplishes the transfer of attention from a percept or action to abstract thought activity, meditation or other forms of creating ASC exert a reverse force. Cognition is inhibited in favor of perception, and the active intellectual style is replaced by a receptive mode. For example, if learning to ride the bike included anxieties about being taught by an impatient father, reliving that experience in a more relaxed state can generalize it, allowing one to view the situation in more forgiving terms.

Some research appears to support this aspect of ASC. One study, for example, presents data showing that as a person enters into a hypnagogic state, the sensory and imagistic worlds become mixed, with approximately half of both being conscious and seemingly real and half being unconscious and seemingly unreal.[21] The processes by which the associations between events and percepts are most easily challenged and changed occur in this state. "The imagery seems to erupt into consciousness from a dissociated subsystem of cognitive control."[22] It may thus appear to us that a memory from the distant past is immediate and real, or that something we are experiencing in the present is actually taking place only in the mind, a daydream rather than a reality. Or the two may be mixed together so that we cannot discern what is memory and what is happening in the immediate present. Most of us have had brief glimpses of such experiences when we have been awakened from a deep sleep by a loud noise.

Several writers have addressed the process of reorientation that takes place in ASC. One of the most fascinating is the account proposed by Nathan Field, who studied the therapeutic function of altered states in the process of psychoanalysis. If he is correct in his assessment of psychoanalysis or psychotherapy in general, the model of altered states would serve all of the major forms of psychological healing. In other words, it is apparently *not* the wisdom of psychoanalytic thought or the logic of psychotherapy models for human behavior that relieves human suffering. It may be merely the *condition* of being in an altered state of consciousness, intentionally or not, that brings about the important bridging into psychological wholeness. Perhaps that is one reason why there are so many different logical systems of counseling that speak to human dynamics. We may build illusory explanations of cause and effect if a psychotherapy patient appears to advance in insight and reason, when actually the real source of healing is inherent in the human psyche, once it is given fertile fields for transcendence.[23]

Other researchers have presented data that suggest that when two or more persons are functioning at a similar state of consciousness, they can have similar or indentical imagery.[24] As a therapeutic event, this can be remarkable in promoting empathy and a sense of understanding between people, certainly between therapist and patient. Sharing an ASC in a therapeutic setting may allow the therapist to understand the inner dynamics of the patient at a deeper level than could be verbalized, making it feasible not only to influence the image of the problem, but also to utilize the power of metaphor at the most profound level. For example, shamans whom I have observed often realize their patients' issues almost instantly through visualization and intuition. They usually spend the rest of the session telling stories or singing songs, ritualizing symbols to reach that deepest imagerial level of understanding. Sometimes they respond almost unconsciously to the patient's internal reality without sensing their physical presence. This is how an ASC can serve as a background that allows for healing to take place.

ASC THROUGH SPACE AND TIME

Throughout history the experience of ASC has played a major role in healing practices around the world. We have just discussed its continued use in the shamanic tradition. The Greek physician Aesclepius, who taught Hippocrates, used the process of "incubation sleep" to induce ASC and reveal cures. The faith cures of Lourdes and other religious rites, mesmeric or even magnetic treatment, all are instances of the induction of an altered state of consciousness.

Physical medical approaches vary from nation to nation; psychological models may not even exist; but whether we are in Japan, Argentina, Germany, Norway, Holland, Mexico, Canada, or the United States, the transpersonal process related to altered states of consciousness is similar or identical. The methods of achieving the state may vary, but in all people who achieve it, the state itself includes a sense of unity and peace. One study compared ten transpersonal healers to determine what, if any, differences exist in their experiences of the healing process. Although five distinct classes of healers were identified, all described processes in which a state of altered consciousness could be recognized. "The results . . . suggest that transpersonal healing/influencing involves the self-regulation of attention, physiology, and cognition, thus inducing altered awareness and reorganizing the healer's construction of cultural and personal realities."[25]

In addition to their applications in healing, altered states of consciousness have always played a major role in bringing new knowledge to the human race. Einstein and Edison are only two examples of people who have explicitly acknowledged the alteration of their states of consciousness as part of their process of making discoveries. In my experience and knowledge of history there have been few, if any, acts of creation in which a state of altered consciousness cannot be inferred as the bridge between conception and action.

Research shows that by shifting to an altered state of consciousness, we can gain access to brain functions ordinarily not available to us in a waking state, providing us with a much broader and richer perspective on any problem. Similar to what we find in REM sleep (the deep dreaming state), the altered state of consciousness that we find in the creative process lifts us out of the strictly linear approach to problem-solving by giving us access to symbols, figures, and feelings. Einstein called this "recombinatory play," meaning that when one is mixing seemingly unrelated elements, allowing them to combine in unexpected ways, surprising new solutions often arise. In the ASC, this "recombinatory play" takes place as the material we ordinarily associate with dreams—symbols, figures, and imagery—begin to mix together. This process has been known for thousands of years, most typically noted in shamanism, where a person might go into an ASC to journey into the dream world, seeking solutions to problems such as where the hunters of his tribe might go to find game, or what herbs might help to heal a sick individual.

RELAXATION AS ASC

Through thirty-minute relaxation sessions, ASC can be induced. One first needs a safe and relaxing environment. Our experience has been that the hospital setting is one of the *least* congenial to any type of conscious relaxation technique. When I was consulting with hypertensive patients in the hospital, I was often called upon to help them relax, either to determine if a therapeutic effect would occur, or to see if relaxation would exacerbate the impact of a prescribed medication. It was always an effort to create an atmosphere conducive to relaxation. There seemed to be a never-ending backdrop of noise: conversation and equipment being moved around or dropped, along with outside noise and activities, including sirens, traffic, and thunderstorms.

In order to contend with the many distractions, I developed an electronic device—simply a small microphone attached to a small amplifier with a pair of earphones—that allowed me to communicate directly to the patient while blocking out the noises around us. This introduced an element of sensory deprivation as well as helping the patient and myself detach ourselves from the hassle around us.

Visual deprivation can be accomplished simply by asking patients to close their eyes. In our hospital work, we used music, drumbeats, ocean wave sounds, wind sounds, and any other acoustical stimulation that would help a person create some altered state of consciousness. The general rule is to find some sound that is ongoing for at least thirty minutes without breaks. It is also important that the music not have words or lyrics, which are distracting.

In his book *The Relaxation Response*, Herbert Benson distilled the relaxation techniques of a thousand years into some very clear and distinct steps.[26] We have used his approach consistently, with remarkable results. Presurgical low-back patients who practiced ten-minute relaxation sessions using our tape-recorded instructions from his book the night before their planned surgeries demonstrated healing times that were twice as fast postsurgery as compared with patients without the preparation, based on the length of their hospital stays.[27] They also needed significantly fewer pain medications and experienced fewer complications. Basically, the steps are as follows:

1. Begin breathing in and out in identical cycles. (I usually count from one to seven with each breath to assure breaths of similar length.

2. After a breathing cycle has been established, only the out-breath need be monitored. A phrase is suggested to help the patient remember to monitor the breathing, as well as to help the process, such as "I am getting better and better," or "I am one."

3. As the breathing is monitored, if any thoughts (especially worries) emerge into consciousness, simply be aware of them, but do not attempt to problem-solve. Merely acknowledge their existence.

We found that the staff of our clinics had to devote some amount of time to the relaxation sessions. It was not enough for the patients to practice merely on their own, because something else almost always took priority over an exercise in which one felt as if nothing was happening. We also went to some effort in creating a proper place for the relaxation sessions to occur, giving the space special features, such as an altar. We found it preferable for the sessions to take place at a carefully chosen, prearranged time each day. This process was helpful for group cohesion, for, as we have already seen, group consciousness can have therapeutic benefits.

THERAPEUTIC USES OF ASC:
SOME PRECAUTIONS

Entering into an altered state of consciousness can be exciting and disturbing at the same time. Those patients who have done it have consistently reported an awareness of many perceptions of various realities available to them. Problems that the patient had been considering in a singular context begin to have multilayered connotations. For example, one man had been quite depressed because he was suffering severe back pain due to an industrial injury and could not return to his beloved job as a steelworker, in which he felt great pride and identification. However, after some experience in an altered state of consciousness, he noted, with some surprise, that he could begin to separate his work-self from his other selves. He could be a "steel-man" inside and do other work outside.

While this particular perceptual shift had a positive outcome, the experience of awakening to the multiple facets of one's personality can be confusing and frightening. Without supportive guidance, the result of the process can be destructive, and I caution those who attempt to have these experiences without supervision. For many people, the exposure to the ASC has been disorienting, threatening their perceptions of the world and often challenging their basic belief systems. When undertaking an ASC as a clinical technique, it is important to have proper support and direction.

It is also important to be cautious when interpreting experiences and symbology associated with ASC sessions, particularly those in which sensational or frightening images are uncovered. Freud discovered that in free association women would describe sexual encounters with their fathers; however, he concluded that these were wishes rather than facts. Perhaps in a similar way many of our patients have interpreted certain ASC images as implying earlier experiences of abuse by a parent or someone else. Many of these individuals did have abusive childhoods in fact, yet this particular symbology also may be derived from other possibilities—a psychological issue of dependency or a need to be loved, a body message of pain (especially when parts of the body most associated with punishment or self-esteem are in stress), a cultural myth of authoritarianism, or even an archetypal process of genetic history. Capture by aliens is another recurrent image in ASC experiences. Regardless of the factual features of these "memories," even if the events really happened, the goal of ASC is not to untangle them, but to uncover resources and paths for transformation. The ultimate benefit of the ASC experience depends on the ability of the patient to activate a plan or insight within her- or himself for positive change. Blaming pain or anxiety on outside events that may or may not have happened years or lifetimes ago only leads to feelings of fear, failure, and isolation.

Whenever ASC is used in a therapeutic setting, it needs to be structured around a sound theory, one with reasonable and acceptable expectations. My own preference is to ground the process in scientific principles. For example, I usually present the process as a function of changing brain patterns, pointing out that the different realities are bringing into awareness other perceptual possibilities. I liken it to changing channels, by which we can see different levels and a broader scope of the same events. Patients usually accept this explanation, at least in the beginning, but once they feel a sense of "realness," often they do not need an explanation—their truth becomes the explanation. In most therapeutic settings it is wise to offer an explanation of this kind and also to have printed material available for patients, their families, and their physicians.

CONCLUSION

Throughout history, a great deal of energy has been invested in achieving some form of altered states of consciousness. In Western culture, we see people turning to alcohol or other drugs in order to fulfill what seems to be a basic need. Perhaps this need arises as a survival instinct, left over from the days in which people who could achieve an ASC were more able to survive. For example, being able to move into other worlds of wisdom enabled the shaman to gain knowledge about the weather and the location of food, as well as providing medicinal aid. (These practices are still going on in some societies, such as the Matses tribe, a subdivision of the Amazon's Mayoruna tribe.)

More consistent with my observations is that perhaps the human need for ASC arises from *pure memory* of a sense of unity and peace that we enjoyed on some plane separate from the ordinary reality of our bodies. The shift to altered states affirms that memory and allows us to return to that consciousness briefly, to feel our connection to the universe and each other. By breaking down the barriers of isolation and individualism, we get in touch with the spiritual side of our souls. Consequently, the practice of entering into altered states of consciousness is a method of reclaiming that sense of universal love and peace, especially when the ordinary reality has become harsh and threatening.

In this chapter, I have tried to present methods for achieving altered states of consciousness that can tap in to the transpersonal realm in ways that are constructive for the individual as well as scientifically acceptable. As we can better recognize the potential of transformation and the conditions that promote healing, perhaps some of the inherent fears of these methods can be channeled into more productive efforts. However, this realm cannot be approached casually. Master teachers and researchers have a great respect for the sacred space of altered states of consciousness, and a real concern is the danger posed by misguided helpers. However, there is no doubt that this particular component of the new era of medicine provides a broad avenue for knowledge and discovery of the healing potential of the human spirit.

‖‖≣‖‖

Interview with Stanley Krippner, PH.D.
Author of *Human Possibilities, The Song of the Siren,* and *The Realms of Healing*

Frank Lawlis: What is your understanding of the altered states of consciousness so often mentioned when we discuss healing?

Stanley Krippner: First, I want to clarify the terminology I will use. *Consciousness* is a word used to describe the pattern of cognitive, perceptual, and emotional functioning of an organism at any point in time. An altered state of consciousness is a shift from that ordinary pattern or function. This will differ from person to person, from culture to culture. Some people walk around in other people's definitions of altered states of consciousness all the time. What is to them an ordinary state would be an altered state to others. So I take a relativistic point of view on the term and how it is used.

A shift from an ordinary state of consciousness can facilitate healing in some cases for a number of reasons. First, it allows access to aspects of the psyche that we do not have in ordinary states—dreams being the obvious examples. There are a lot of dreams in which information comes to the person for healing—herbs, exercises, and the like. It is remarkable how specific the dreams can be. Second, in an altered state, we may have a different self-image; self-image is very important in healing. Some people may see themselves as chronically ill. When they go into an altered state, for the first time they might realize that they can think of themselves as a well person. Sometimes meditation helps people drop a negative self-image, after which they feel that they can choose a different one.

A third reason that altered states of consciousness help in healing processes is that they shift patterns of thinking and feeling. Often people get stuck in a rational, analytical mode of thought that is not helping them get better. But in altered states they may have more access to emotions and their personal myths; this shift in patterns can aid in more balance and better health. The fourth reason is that sometimes altered states can serve as an adjunct to other forms of healing, such as surgery. This is obvious: one would not undergo surgery in an ordinary state of consciousness.

FL: Do you believe that there are multiple levels of consciousness?

SK: Yes. This is relevant to the third reason that I discussed, that we have different patterns of thinking and feeling in altered states than we do in ordinary states. Sometimes these differences are so profound that we might slip into a subpersonality. In multiple personalities, there are possibilities of realizing healthier dimensions, and within a few minutes a person can slip out of their diseased condition. This remarkable feat demonstrates the human capacity to heal. I am not saying that we should create altered personalities for healing, but that we should use this information to show what is possible.

FL: Is there a shadow side to this process?

SK: There are destructive subpersonalities, yes. An important principle is that as someone who is trying to facilitate healing, one does not impose one's own images onto another person. If you superimpose your own imagery, you might be feeding into a symbol system that is just the opposite of what it is for you. For you, the snake may be a healing symbol of transformation; for others, the snake might be a symbol of something poisonous. People need to use altered states with a great deal of care and concern to avoid bringing out a destructive or shadow personality in someone else.

FL: Do you believe that drug-induced changes in consciousness are the same as changes that occur through other means?

SK: No, they are different. Some are better for some problems than others. People respond differently to different means of induction. Drumming and meditation are safer than drug-induced states, but certainly with a well-trained therapist or shaman, drug-induced states can be helpful. My opinion on this differs from those of many others in the field in that I feel that information gained from drug experiences can provide possibilities for growth without the continued use of the substance. I do not recommend a lot of drug use, unless it is part of the culture in which a person is raised. A drug-induced state should be used only for a sense of direction, to be worked with without drugs over a longer period of time.

FL: Across cultures, do you see consistency in the use of altered states of consciousness?

SK: No, there is a lot of inconsistency. In the first place, anthropologists have observed that 89 percent of all cultures have a socially approved method of altering consciousness—drugs, drumming, dancing, meditation. We lack that in Western cultures, except for alcohol and tobacco, and we are really missing out on the value of altered states as a healing tool. There is always an uphill resistance to the use of altered states in medicine—hypnosis, dream analysis, and so on, but we need to persist in this regard.

I think that achieving altered states of consciousness may be a human need in terms of acquiring wisdom, enhancing creativity, or even just having fun. People feel a hunger for something deeper than their ordinary state of consciousness. That is one of the reasons for the popularity of rock music, even rap music. That repetitive beat brings about consciousness change, not unike what happens in religious revival meetings. These doors out of our traditional ways of behaving enable us to get fresh and new perspectives. In this regard, industrialized cultures are quite poverty-stricken compared with indigenous cultures. These processes are valuable in terms of cultural and individual well-being.

⫴ 6 ⫴

IMAGERY

The Power of the Symbol

B OB WAS A PATIENT with the diagnosis of multiple myeloma who
had come to us in search of possible avenues for his disease management. He was on chemotherapy and under an oncologist's care;
based on lab reports of his protein count, the disease was active and
progressive. Multiple myeloma is a type of cancer that involves the
manufacture of malformed stem and plasma cells in the bone marrow
that, if allowed to grow, will damage healthy cells and create massive
circulatory problems. The bones will begin to break down, causing
severe pain. In most cases the disease is terminal.

Bob was an energetic and curious man who had enjoyed a long career as a banker; however, he had recently retired to spend the rest of
his life on a farm. He expressed some regret at this change, but he was
hoping to adjust well to his new life.

We taught Bob a form of voluntary relaxation in which he would
progressively relax muscle groups throughout his body, beginning with
his feet and working all the way up through his legs, pelvis, trunk,
chest, arms, back, neck, and face. In this deeply relaxed state, there are
dramatic changes in the brain waves that allow the person to become
open and receptive to suggestions of imagery.

During the state of deep relaxation Bob began to focus on a visual image of the cancer cells. What he wanted to see was a black, ugly monster with tentacles; however, what actually emerged were very small human-looking organisms that were working very hard. When I asked what they were doing, he replied that they were bank tellers who were trying to balance the accounts for the end of the day. After some discussion of the implications of that image, he determined that the cancer was a series of mistaken account papers that were clogging up the whole system, and that if things did not clear up soon, the system would never balance. In many ways, the cancer represented waste and carelessness that was complicated by the computer; without a careful analysis, the problems would be extended to the next banking day, the next quarter, the next fiscal year, and so on.

At this point Bob felt that he had reached a place of clarification, and he left the office with a sense of direction. His plan was to focus upon forgiving himself and resolving the confusion of his life. He wanted to instigate a "simpler" way of life by beginning to balance the credits and debits.

Bob returned to my office in three weeks, disappointed and frustrated. The results of his lab tests had not changed, and he was feeling desperate. In spite of his goals, he had found himself bored on the farm with the "simple" approach to life. He continued to read banking journals and to contemplate various economic issues with the same interest as before, but now he felt guilty about doing it. And when practicing his imagery, he saw that the "tellers were still falling behind."

We began the imagery process again. His cancer imagery was the same as before, with the mistakes and incorrect audits compounding the problem, but we now progressed to the next step, imagining the immunity process, the white blood cells, at work. In a fairly complicated, yet physiologically correct, metaphor, Bob saw three types of white blood cells, the "janitors," the "personnel managers" and the "audit-trainers." The janitors were the cells who cleaned up the mess. As trash accumulated, they immediately moved in to keep the office clean. The personnel managers served two functions—to reduce stress on the tellers and to oversee the production of accounting. They would support the tellers in their performance of the tasks, and they would also manage their general energy level. For example, they would restrict the number of customers or the number of working hours to just the right level so that the tellers would not overwork. Bob taught them breathing exercises, posture, and pacing, as well as practical accounting approaches to reduce errors. The audit-trainers also helped in the reduction of errors by supervising the ongoing accounting process and allowing the tellers to relax while they audited the accounts.

I have never worked in a bank, so I am ignorant of the various tasks involved, but all of this made sense to Bob. The roles he described also made sense to me in terms of the white blood cell processes. The janitors were acting like phagocytes, scavengers of waste and other enemies of the body such as malformed cells, used-up red blood cells, and the like. The personnel managers could be seen as T cells who manage the attacks on cancer cells but who also serve to reduce the attack when appropriate. They are very sensitive to the energy level of the host. The audit-trainers appeared to me to be similar to the B cells, a sophisticated educator-type that helps determine what disease is and what it is not. They have good memories for past disease types and can relate this information to other cells for action. They are the ones that keep us from getting the measles or mumps over and over again.

Bob made another important decision in his life: he returned to his job in the banking business. His imagery practice had stimulated him to think of new management techniques. He had also come to the conclusion that his banking career gave him pleasure. If he might die in the coming year anyway, he would rather be in a bank than anywhere else.

Bob returned to his job, his cancer moved into remission, and last I heard he was happy and still clear of disease. Although it is impossible to assign a cause-and-effect connection to a specific case, one can only wonder: What function did the imagery have? Was the image the path, the pathfinder, or did it have nothing to do with the remission of the disease?

What Is Imagery?

We are constantly creating images simply by virtue of the normal, everyday process by which our minds organize sensory input from the world around us. For example, the wave forms we call "sound" stimulate special nerve fibers that convey some association to the brain, by which an auditory image that we recognize is formed. Visual stimulation is organized into forms that are associated with specific objects we can label. The "image" is basically the entity that our consciousness formulates as the result of sensory and memory processes.

Mental imagery is not always dependent on outside stimuli, however. The proof of this is found in our dreams, daydreams, and imaginations. Consider a poet or novelist, for instance, who is able to consciously create vivid imagery and even characterizations of people that are convincing in terms of how they match up with external reality. In this case, it is almost as if the imagery process is running in reverse, with the image beginning in the mind and moving outward into the world to create an external framework or model of reality. In other words, through using imagery we can create mental models that we then use to guide the way we live or the way we experience our lives.

Since the initial studies of imagery and its healing effects on the mind and body were undertaken, more specific definitions of imagery have emerged, broadening our idea of what it means to create a mental image. For instance, rather than limit it to the visual, we can associate imagery with one or more of the other senses: hearing, smelling, touching, tasting, and feeling.

For example, visual imagery arises from the ability to "see" entities or events—a tree, a childhood birthday party—without the assistance of actual external stimulation. Although much literature in the field of imagery uses "imagery" and "visual imagery" interchangeably, I have found that at least forty percent of the patients with whom I work cannot "see things" with their eyes closed. These people become justifiably frustrated if they are asked to visualize their bodies or a scene. They also have some difficulty going on "inner journeys" if only visual cues are given.

In my research I have found that auditory imagination—the ability to hear things without external stimulation—is the next most frequently available ability and is as effective as visual imagination in the healing process. For example, most people can imagine the sound of their mother calling them by name, or the melody and words of a favorite song.

Olfactory imagery has great emotional power, perhaps because the olfactory center of the brain is close to the emotional center or because there are significantly fewer nerve conjunctions in the smell process as compared with the other senses. If a person can imagine the smell of bread baking or bacon cooking, or recall the smell of a lover, a powerful emotional context arises. Closely associated with smell, of course, is taste, yet imagining the taste of chocolate or fruit does not appear to stimulate as powerful an emotional response as imagining a smell.

Of all the kinds of imagery, touch imagery evokes the greatest variety of responses, depending on the individual's personal history. For example, a person who was physically abused as a child, and who has done no healing around that experience, may become frightened or defensive at even the suggestion of being touched. By contrast, a person who is comfortable with his or her body and sensuality may feel blissful and strong when the imagery involves being touched by another person. Many things about a person can be discovered through touch or the suggestion of touch as evoked through imagery, whether it be associations of being punished, being comforted, being sexually mistreated, or having trustful and affectionate sensual experiences.

The most powerful imagery for people suffering from chronic pain is kinesthetic in nature, that is, involving the matrix of feelings associated with muscular stresses and tensions, actual physical touch, and physical movements that occur with breathing, dancing, singing, speaking, sports activities, and the like. Within each of us is a proprioceptive system that interprets and coordinates all movements, tensions, and stresses within the body. It helps us coordinate our efforts in running, standing, sitting down, and so on. Kinesthetic experiences are dependent on proprioceptive faculties of our bodymind. The best example of this might be the pleasure we derive from dancing or playing a sport.

A mistake many therapists make is to assume that only visual imagery has a significant impact on the body. They may find that having patients only visualize their blood vessels becoming more relaxed brings about no measurable change in the blood pressure. However, asking patients to feel their heart relaxing, slowing down, radiating warmth out to their hands and feet as they picture themselves moving slowly around a warm, crackling campfire on a summer beach, might evoke a full kinesthetic range of experience, and the blood pressure normalizes.

MEMORY IMAGERY VERSUS FANTASY IMAGERY

Although the sensory mode is useful in determining how best to induce imagery for healing, it is also important to look at the difference between fantasy and memory-induced imagery. Memory imagery is the ability to reexperience an event that occurred in the past. For example, when I taught airline pilots how to reduce their blood pressure, I first asked them to find an event in their past that was associated with comfort and relaxation. Their most typical memories in this regard were of being sung to or rocked as small children.

The sensory input called into play through memory may include moving, hearing, smelling, and touching. As the airline pilots began reliving their memories, their blood pressure was electronically monitored to determine the effects of their imagery. Any other physiological changes were similarly measured, and we carefully noted which memories induced which changes. We discovered that exploring memories along with monitoring physiological functions is an excellent first step in designing effective imagery.

Fantasy imagery is different from memory imagery in that we are imagining what we have never experienced. While portions of fantasy may be drawn from experiences we've had in real life, other portions may be quite outside our range of experience. The mind is able to blend these together, though the mechanism that makes this happen is still a mystery to researchers. For example, one might fantasize having a sexual encounter with a famous movie star, with such strong imagery that it produces measurable physical responses, such as penile erection and other muscular and glandular reactions. While the physcial responses may be drawn from real-life experiences, the specific encounter with the movie star is not.

It takes time and energy to manufacture the various components of any fantasy, since fantasy does not, like memory, simply pop into our minds from the past with an orchestrated physiological and psychological response. The difficulty with integrating the various components may have more to do with limits we place on ourselves as adults than it does with anything physiological. Children, on the other hand, respond extremely well to fantasy stories, especially when they involve space trips, adventures to faraway places, and animals. One theory is that children have only thin boundaries between imagination and ordinary reality, and they relate quickly to suggestions involving extraordinary reality. By contrast, most of us, by the time we are adults, have learned how to discriminate between fantasy and reality, and we have been conditioned by society to spend as little time as possible in the former realm.

INTERVENTION IMAGERY VERSUS DIAGNOSIS IMAGERY

The notion that imagery could be used as a diagnostic tool appears to be accepted even in the medical community. For example, Vert Mooney published the method of the pain drawing as a means for determining the degree of pain suffered by low-back-pain patients; he found this method to be highly reliable and predictable.[1] Later work aimed at evaluating imagery drawings has led to an imagery system that has now become a primary objective tool for determining outcomes for surgical, pharmaceutical, and pain-management programs.[2]

Although intervention imagery has not won complete acceptance in psychological research, the medical community has quickly adopted diagnostic imagery protocols. Imagery drawing techniques for headaches, arthritis, obesity, and cancer appear to be commonplace now, both as diagnostic tools and as aids in patient education and communication. Information about the patient's perceptions of his or her physical aspects greatly benefits the patient and helps the health professional diagnose a variety of conditions and evaluate the outcome of treatment. What the disease means in the patient's life is also communicated through the imagery. For example, for obsessively self-reliant persons, debilitating illness or chronic pain could be devastating, seeming to rob them of everything they value. By contrast, very dependent people might actually find some sense of security in having an illness, since it would guarantee that others would have to take care of them. Either tendency would be revealed in diagnostic imagery work.

Diagnostic imagery can lead to a much closer relationship between the physician or health care professional and the patient, resulting in both a better understanding of the problem and greater compliance in terms of the patient's following a prescribed course of treatment. For example, by examining the pain drawings of a person with low back pain, it is relatively easy to evaluate the imagery for the emotional basis of the pain and to identify which portions of the brain or nervous system are affected. The level of the patient's pain tolerance can also be determined accurately. An effective treatment protocol can then be outlined.

The intervention model of imagery—that if one changes an image of one's disease or problem, the physical components will change accordingly—is controversial. This theory would have it that if we can make ourselves ill by stressful imagery, then we can make ourselves well using imagery that is more positive. Evidence and clinical experience do support the idea that modifying imagery that causes anxiety or inaccurate expectations can help also reduce complications in the healing process. The field of sports psychology provides many examples. For instance, someone who has the image of him- or herself as a loser, a second-class athlete, can often reach a fuller performance potential by changing that image. Similarly, most Olympic-class athletic training now includes having athletes mentally rehearse their physical performance, resulting in significant, measurable improvements in the actual performance. By the same token, studies that relate immune deficiency to grief or depression support the fact that stressful imagery has an impact on physical and mental capacities.

The greatest support for intervention imagery as a means of enhancing capacity is related to this "mental rehearsal" process. Just as in sports psychology, a person mentally plays out an upcoming event; for instance, one might mentally rehearse coping mechanisms one finds effective for dealing with the particular medical issue one is facing. Along these lines, Achterberg and Kenner developed a mental rehearsal for burn patients in preparation for therapy, using relaxation coping strategies in the imaged event.[3] The results were dramatic, indicating that these patients experienced significantly less pain and anxiety than those who went into the therapy without mental rehearsal. Another research study demonstrated reduced nausea and vomiting with a similar protocol for cancer patients undergoing chemotherapy.[4]

There are many case studies of individuals who appear to have changed the direction of their diseases by using imagery, such as the case described at the beginning of this chapter. However, the process is complex because imagery practice includes a totality of emotions, lifestyle issues, relationships, and values. A peaceful, nonaggressive person may feel challenged and threatened by the effort to image sharks or white knights. Because it is important that the imagery and the patient's belief system be compatible, the effectiveness of one image or another is a highly individual issue, making it particularly difficult to design research studies around the relationship between intervention imagery and health.

IMAGERY AS A PREDICTIVE TOOL

In a recent issue of the *New England Journal of Medicine* on alternative methods of cancer care, imagery was listed among the top four most frequently used techniques by patients.[5] Using imagery to identify and focus a person's goals or intentions around healing or combating a challenging illness or injury is now routinely discussed in medical circles in the context of hypnosis, altered states of consciousness, and sports psychology.

However, when Jeanne Achterberg and I first began exploring the relationships between imagery and physiological functions in the early 1970s, there was very little support available for our research. Medical experts were still denying that there was any link between stress and disease. When I visited the American Heart Association in Dallas at that time, the person guiding me through the offices remarked that the association was not willing to acknowledge any link between psychological state and heart disease, and that there were serious doubts that anyone in the organization would publish such "unfounded opinions." We were met with a similar rebuff from the American Cancer Society.

There have been, of course, some rather dramatic reversals of this attitude even in the past five years.

Science begins as the observation of nature. The method of scientific observation might be termed correlational because one is attempting to establish a direct link between one event and another. Scientific literature is filled with experiments using a statistical basis to establish correlations between a seemingly infinite number of phenomena. My own and Dr. Achterberg's first approaches to imagery and human physiology were also correlational in nature, as we attempted to see how psychological and imagerial content would relate to disease functions.

Our first study of the possible impact of imagery on physical functions and disease included cancer patients under the care of Dr. Carl Simonton, an oncologist. Since they were already participating in imagery and counseling as part of a psychosocial program, Dr. Simonton's patients represented a homogeneous group of individuals for our project. The study required patients to have blood tests taken regularly and to undergo various psychological tests. To stay in the program, patients also had to be committed to these efforts.

The results were revealing. Using a standardized method for evaluating the imagery, we were able to predict with 92 percent accuracy what any patient's health picture would be in two months. In parallel, it was shown that lab tests could not accurately predict the course of a disease. One conclusion we drew from this study is that a patient's psychological outlook, determination, and belief that he or she will get well tell us more about his or her chances of surviving a disease like cancer than does anything we can measure in the lab.

While Dr. Achterberg and I felt that we were at the cutting edge of a medical breakthrough, when we attempted to publish this research, medical journal editors refused to accept our findings, primarily because the results were not believable according to established patterns of thinking. We finally published the studies in a statistical journal called *Multivariate Clinical Experimental Research*, because the editorial review was interested in our methodology and interpretation from a statistical perspective; the clinical results of the study were secondary.[6] The fact that psychological states could predict cancer survival rates might not have been in alignment with their belief system, but the magnitude of our numbers and the level of sophistication in our study of them intrigued the editors.

We then became the chief evaluators for the Comprehensive Cancer Care Program sponsored by the National Cancer Institute at the University of Texas Health Science Center in Dallas, where we had a very different population to study. Here, our group was made up of primarily indigent, minority patients who had no idea of the imagery process. Nevertheless, our study once again proved imagery to be an extremely powerful predictor, especially in regard to rehabilitation efforts and quality of life for the patients.[7] In another project conducted at the University of Texas Health Science Center in San Antonio involving throat cancer patients, we found that the imagery measures were highly related to rehabilitation success as well as to survival and were superior to medical measures of disease severity or process.[8]

EXPERIMENTAL STUDIES
WITH CONSCIOUS INTENTION

As scientific observations continue to support hypotheses of cause-and-effect correlations between conscious intent and imagery, health researchers continue to look for ways to use the mind in healing. John Schneider provided a significant study in the field of imagery intervention and psychoneuroimmunology.[9] Both the design of the study and its results were profound. Focusing on a particular white blood cell (neutrophil), Schneider demonstrated that college students could use imagery to control the locations and behaviors of their immunity elements. This study paved the way for other research involving neutrophils, one of which showed that not only were the behaviors of neutrophils related to stress, but effectiveness in their abilities to find and destroy toxic substances was directly enhanced through imagery and relaxation. A broad array of dissertations then emerged from the University of North Texas psychology department, revealing a variety of ways that imagery can control various immunity processes. One of these studies measured secretory IgA (Immunoglobulin A), a substance found in saliva that is associated with immunity.[10] This substance is important in such studies because the amount present in the saliva is a dependable measure of how the immune system is working. Another study demonstrated that not only could immunity components be affected by imagery, but certain types of cells in the immune system could be controlled with a surprising degree of discrimination.[11] These researchers instructed their subjects to image lymphocytes or neutrophils. The results indicated that the cells responded to imagery that the people created in their minds, and that the imagery could be designed in such a way as to discriminate between the two types of cells.

While the research clearly demonstrated that people could affect the production and behavior of components in the immune system through imagery, it was yet to be demonstrated that such abilities could help to heal a person who was actually ill. However, the research evidence continues to grow, showing that a patient's imaging can have a positive influence on the healing process in such conditions as pruritic eczema,[12] acne vulgaris,[13] birth pain,[14] diabetes,[15] breast cancer,[16] arthritis,[17] migraine and tension headaches,[18] and treatment of severe burns.[19] The overall conclusions are that conscious intent can be effective in the healing process for some patients, depending on their personal beliefs and characteristics, as well as the psychosocial environment in which the work is conducted. Some of these factors are discussed in our examination of the therapeutic considerations of conscious intent.

As the technology for measuring immediate responses to imagery becomes more sophisticated, our understanding of the body-mind-spirit interactions can be better appreciated. Achterberg, for example, described a case study of a patient who was imaging a process of kidney healing while being evaluated by the BEAM (Brain Electrical Activity Map).[20] The patient's pre-imagery brain scan shows a concentration of activity in the cortex; however, after an imaging session the BEAM measured a dramatic change, with activity spreading throughout every area of the brain. This measure shows that there are significant differences between what portions of the brain are activated by ordinary reality and those involved in imaging. The findings in this observation were also consistent with research exploring the healing mechanisms using altered states of consciousness.

Perhaps the most exciting development relating to imagery has been the discovery of microtubules within the nerve cell structure itself.[21] Microtubules serve as the skeleton of the nerve cell, by which the cell maintains its integrity. We now know that these structures vibrate with information and create a second order of communication from one cell to another. At last, we have evidence that helps explain a new paradigm of consciousness that goes beyond the old electrical model of nerve conduction, whereby messages between cells are sent from brain to cell and back again via a system that resembles a complex telephone network. This old model was never fully able to account for the multiple messages that occur within consciousness nor for the dramatically widespread impact of imagery.

This new model of the neurological system allows us to begin developing a far broader and more sophisticated model of how healing—and particularly imagery healing—takes place. For example, it can be surmised that a particular image may set up vibrational responses that send out waves of information, communicating much more powerfully and effectively than with only a direct stimulation at a nerve ending. The old model might be compared to communicating a message to a million people by speaking to one person at a time, while the new model is more like communicating to the same number of people simultaneously by broadcasting the message with radio waves.

Imagery and intent have been used in healing for thousands of years, perhaps since the beginning of humankind. Yet, perhaps because their secrets remain hidden from us due to our own limited understanding of the relationship between consciousness and the body, their widespread acceptance in modern medicine has been slow in coming. Their use requires time, sensitivity, and specialized training that isn't included in the education of physicians. In many instances, introducing them goes beyond the parameters of today's health care system. For these reasons, they may continue to be considered only a complementary form of therapy, which individual patients will have to seek out on their own.

Therapeutic Use of Intervention Imagery

Like most applications to medical problems, there is a method to conscious intent, at least in terms of intervention imagery approaches. The four primary phases related to using intervention imagery in therapy are:

imagery of the problem
imagery of internal resources
imagery of external resources
imagery enhancement

Imagery of the problem generally begins with "facing the enemy." What this means is carefully analyzing the problem, with a minimum of anxiety or fear. For example, although the thought of cancer invokes stress, it is very helpful to examine the patient's perception of cancer through imagery. With relaxation as a prelude, the patient is led into the careful and thoughtful determination of what dimensions are inherent in the problem.

There are several questions the therapist can ask at this point in order to help the patient in his or her exploration of the problem:

- If you could see the problem, what would it look like? What colors would be apparent? What special characteristics are there?
- If you could hear the problem, what would it be saying? Does it have anything to say to you or to anyone else?
- If you could hold it or touch it, what would it feel like? Is it warm or cold? Does it feel good? Bad?
- If you could smell it, what would it smell like?
- As far as you can tell, does the problem have a personality? Does it have emotions like anger, sadness, fear, happiness?
- Does the problem have a reason for being? What are its motivations, its intentions? Does it have a plan?
- Everything has a weakness or vulnerability. Can you see

what the weakness of the problem is? How would you
weaken or destroy the problem, if you wanted to?

In Bob's story, you'll recall, he began to depict his cancer as bank
tellers whose accounts wouldn't balance, and he felt that if he were
there to help he could get things back on track. While it is only one
part of an effective therapy plan, the purpose of the imagery is to help
the individual recognize his or her emotional response to the problem.
In this way, it is often possible to identify and resolve attitudinal issues
that might otherwise impede the healing process. For example, I have
found that there is often a direct relationship between pain and self-
image. We usually have some memory of pain as part of learning to
grow up. The pain of punishment, for instance, implied that we were
bad. Therefore, when we image a source of pain there is always the
possibility that we will regard the pain and any illness associated with
it as punishment. It is quite common for guilt and fear to arise with
this association, which can result in a person unconsciously sabotaging
the imaging process. For the patient to reach some understanding of
his or her self-image and how the pain affects it is important.

There are three important characteristics to consider in the imagery
of a problem: the clarity of the problem, its strength, and its power or
vulnerability. First, how clearly and concretely is the problem perceived by the patient? For example, if the person can only vaguely
describe it, picturing it as, for example, "a big black cloud hanging
over my life," there is less clarity than if he or she is able to describe
it, as Bob did, in terms as specific as bank tellers unable to balance
their accounts.

Second, how much strength does the problem have? Does the patient picture his or her pain or illness as totally overwhelming, as an
annoying presence, or as a minor inconvenience? In most cases, this
consideration involves the issue of control—how much control of his
or her own life the patient may be losing to the disease. Control covers
a broad range. Some problems, though they can't be controlled, can
be ignored or avoided without vastly compromising the person's quality of life. For example, we might not be able to change or control an
alcoholic parent's behavior, but we can prevent it from controlling our

own life. Similarly, alcoholism may not be seen as a "controllable disease," but through community support it can be managed. These are all questions we would categorize under "strength" in designing an imaging program for a patient.

Third is the power or vulnerability factor. Inherent in this consideration is the perception that there is an intelligence or purpose that the problem seems to possess. For instance, the cancer or pain may seem to have the intent of consuming the patient or even to be part of a larger strategy for accomplishing this. It would be important to know what the person's image is of how that might work. Sometimes our picture of a disease entity's process can be aligned with how that entity actually operates. For example, the AIDS virus has a kind of intelligence that directs it to invade the T4 cells, taking up residence within them and using the cells themselves to help it reproduce. With this picture in mind, a person might design imagery of the T4 cells as building up resistance, setting limits, and not allowing the AIDS virus to enter.

Once we have a complete understanding of the imagery involved in the problem, we can help the patient move on to developing imagery of his internal resources—what he has in the way of capacities for combating or healing a disease or injury. Patient education is very important at this point, especially when it comes to discussing the nature of the disease. Basically the same questions are again addressed:

- What do your internal resources look like? Do they have a color? How big are they? How many of them can you see?
- Can you hear them? What are they saying or singing? Do they have a message for you? Do they have a message for the problem?
- If you could touch them, what would they feel like? Are they strong? Are they hot or cold? Do they have a personality? Are there emotions, like anger, happiness, sadness? Intelligence? Is there a strategy for coping with the problem? Is there a master plan, an organizational plan, a person in charge?

Patients may have a clear image of their internal resources, but most often they do not. To assist them in developing their imagery, I often spend some time describing their internal healing resources, and what they need to accomplish, sometimes in physiological terms but often using metaphors to simplify more complex physiological mechanisms.

For instance, I might explain how their bodies have the capacity to produce endorphine pain managers on their own and what they can do to stimulate their production. Or I might quickly describe how their hormonal systems affect their emotions, and vice versa, and how certain brain functions cause mood changes, and so on. On occasion we use cartoon characters to describe the natural healing process after surgery, such as the way skin grafts work, how bone grows and heals, how tissue repairs itself, or how cardiovascular repair mechanisms grow new components. When patients have a clear picture of what's going on with their bodies and what they can do to encourage a normal healing response, the imagery they initiate tends to be much more effective.

It is interesting to note that when the therapist uses metaphor to describe a complex physiological process, patients usually use it as a springboard for developing imagery and symbols from their own lives, as Bob did with his banking experience. This "personalization" of the imagery is what we call the empowerment phase. When people can create imagery with their own power icons and dynamics that they understand and trust, the physiological process is likely to progress.

The external resources are any allies outside ourselves that we might rally to our cause. Examples of such resources might include a physician's knowledge and skill with drugs and surgery, diet, friends and family, the sun, exercise, and one's work environment. We usually request that patients work with the image of a "health pie," which they partition into the various resources available to them. In the process, they indicate the degree of importance that each of the "slices" holds. For example, if a patient places fifty percent of his or her faith in chemotherapy to eradicate a tumor, he or she allocates half the pie to that treatment. The health professional can then join the patient in emphasizing this healing technique in the treatment.

The fourth step in imagery therapy is to further enhance the healing intensity by honoring the process. To do this we help integrate the imagery into the patient's lifestyle and worldview. A daily routine of ritual is prescribed at this point, with extra care taken to make certain the symbols of the imagery really come from the patient's own inner world. Songs and music that energize the patient are played once or twice a day. If physicial exercise appears to enhance the positive aspects of healing, it is included in the daily regimen as well.

Artwork, such as drawings and sculpture, can be displayed in the patient's home or office as a reminder of personal healing imagery. For example, one woman had a large collection of frog figures, some carved, some shaped of clay or other materials. To her, frogs meant change and transformation, and looking at the little figures enhanced her healing process, which included inner and outer transformation. The frog was also an important symbol in her imagery.

If color is important to patients, I recommend that they paint at least one room in their home to attune them with the colors of their imagery work. The colors and patterns in bed sheets, slipcovers, and clothes can also help create a healing environment. The point is that whatever symbology appears in the person's healing imagery can be brought into everyday reality so that he or she can bring the imagery alive in the most powerful way possible.

Enchancement techniques to help crystallize the symbolism can be as innovative as the therapist and patient. The most immediate effect is that the enhancement helps frame the image in terms of the person's everyday experience. The imagery process, in other words, becomes integrated with the person's day-to-day life rather than being set apart as something special.

Biofeedback technology has been an invaluable tool for helping people develop imagery that actually affects them on a physiological level. For example, if someone is using the symbol of white light to produce a calming effect to reduce hypertension, biofeedback allows that individual to refine the imagery until it produces the desired physiological changes.

By having the patient sit in front of a machine with a light, meter, or screen that indicates changes in the patient's vital signs and having that person experiment with different imagery, the therapist can quickly determine whether that imagery is producing the desired effect. Generally speaking, we find that one or more of the following changes can deepen the effect of the imagery:

1. Changes in the breathing pattern
2. Humming different tones for long periods
3. Using personal chants
4. Singing or listening to music
5. Assuming different postures
6. Visualizing different scenes
7. Viewing or remembering anatomical pictures or educational material
8. Using animal characters
9. Visualizing colors within body parts
10. Moving the body to symbolize the understanding of disease and healing (such as "dancing" the white blood cells)

The body and spirit do not communicate in words, but through symbols and subtle configurations of experienced associations and information. For example, an expert cannot, by looking only at physiological cues such as heart rate and breathing, distinguish whether someone is experiencing fear or joy. Both of these emotions produce elevated rates in many physiological areas. For this reason, it is important to learn something about what moves a patient emotionally and spiritually. Is the elevated heart rate that we see when we mention standing on a mountain the result of fear, because the patient is afraid of heights? Or is the elevated heart rate the result of feeling inspired by the beautiful view? Asking someone to describe what is going on emotionally when we see dramatic changes in biofeedback measurements can be critical, providing us with solid cues for helping the person create imagery that "speaks" to him or her at a deep level.

As we get to know the symbols that most dramatically affect our lives or the lives of our patients, we go beyond technique and move into self-discovery. We begin to see that the symbols and imagery that produce physiological changes also reveal a good deal about who we are—about how we experience our lives and make decisions. With

Bob, for example, it became clear that banking was his life. Symbols such as the bank tellers' problems spoke to him directly because they were actually drawn from meaningful life experience.

It is interesting to note that guided imagery practice includes the four components of ritual, which we have already discussed. First, we assume a higher realm of wisdom than our own. In this way, we often move outside our ordinary reality or realm of awareness, passing through a transitional stage where we begin to identify with new values or perceptions about our lives. Finally, we integrate these changes back into ordinary life.

THE POWER OF SYMBOLS TO HEAL

Whatever the meaning the imagery components convey to the patient, and whatever his or her apparent understanding of them happens to be, the most powerfully affecting symbols represent a source of considerable energy and potential for change. When assessing which symbols to work with, it is important to find out what symbols are more powerful than others for the individual. Is there an inherent force within an image—such as a cross or a serpent—that makes it particularly potent for him or her? Historically, nations and groups have drawn power from such symbols, displaying them on flags and shields. Businesses employ specialists to create logos, using such symbols for the enhancement of good fortune. These examples suggest to us that certain imagery is far more than mere decoration.

From what inner resources do these symbols derive? Achterberg has presented seven probable sources of images:[22]

1. *Neurological hardwire response* refers to the "hardwiring" of the brain. By touching certain portions of the brain with low-level electrical current, we can cause a person to perceive lights, geometric figures, sounds. Similar perceptions can be produced by chemicals such as LSD or other hallucinogenic substances. Basically four symbols occur: spirals, webs, lattices, and geometric figures.

2. *Mind-body communication.* The communications between mind and body are such that we often get a sense of an impending illness. For example, before an outward symptom appears, our body may recognize

subtle sensory input associated with a disease state and then communicate it to the mind as a vague anxiety or fear. There is also evidence that in an ASC we can gain access to the early imagery of a disease. For example, research has shown that the imagery in pictures drawn by cancer patients often depicts evidence of the disease progressing long before that fact is revealed by medical tests.

3. *Psychological dynamics.* The largest body of information about the altered state of consciousness and the production of imagery and symbols is found in the psychoanalytic literature. With this literature, however, there is the general attitude that the imagery is the result of individual "dream language" produced by the patient's conflicts and fears. Within this perspective, we tend to regard imagery of this kind as being relevant only to that individual, though of course there are schools of thought that suggest that some dream imagery is universal.

4. *Nature.* For those who live very close to nature, such as early aboriginal peoples, there is often an acute awareness of the natural elements—wind, lightning, earthquakes, and volcanic eruptions, to say nothing of the changes of the seasons and the shifting of the moon, stars, and sun. The unconscious might note and store the subtle clues (changes in barometric pressure, ionization of the air, and the like) produced by nature long before a storm, earthquake, or other natural phenomenon occurs. While the person might not have conscious awareness of these early clues, he or she might gain access to them through entering an altered state of consciousness, as appears to be the case in many shamanic traditions.

Some imagery may actually be generated within Mother Earth. For example, in directing spiritual pilgrimages across land sites that have been used in ancient ritual healing, I have observed that when we induce a receptive state of consciousness (through drumming, gonging, or sitting in silence), consistent imagery emerges across the group. For example, as we explored sites in Ireland, I set up a quasi-experimental situation in which I asked each of some thirty participants to compare their imagery after being at a particular place. The consistency was amazing.

5. *Culture.* A great deal of our imagery arises from the culture in which we live; different cultures assign different values to different

objects. For example, in one culture a snake might symbolize wisdom and healing; in another it might be the symbol of evil. In one culture a feather might have a high symbolic value; in another the feather might be meaningless, but a car might be a powerful image.

6. *Collective unconscious.* Carl Jung proposed that in addition to the individual unconscious, there is a collective unconscious whose imagery and symbols derive from the experiences of the human race as a whole. The speculation is that we may receive some of this information genetically but that much of it exists as a kind of external pool of consciousness that has a life of its own. Through entering an altered state of consciousness, we can sometimes gain access to this pool, usually in the form of symbols and imagery.

7. *Pure symbols.* The most controversial source of symbology for academic scientists is the material that might be derived from the collective unconscious or from "pure" sources. The pure source is that broader scope of symbols that may encompass the past and future sources as indicators or maps of the evolution of humankind. These may be inherent within our consciousness as a means of promoting evolution and progression of spirit—karma or the process of soul development. Many of these conceptual ideas are reiterated in Joseph Campbell's work about mythic journeys and cross-cultural consistencies. Some of the most common are the creation, birth/rebirth, the flood, search for the beloved, search for the Grail, and search for God.

In her book *Signs of Life*, Angeles Arrien points to five symbols—the cross, spiral, circle, square and triangle—that appear to carry similar meanings across cultures and time.[23] She interprets the cross to symbolize a focus on interpersonal relationships, and the spiral to symbolize transformation. The circle represents the underlying dimension of unity and individuation; the square, a person's involvement in community; and the triangle, an attention to higher aspirations and goals.

Interestingly, the pure symbols of Arrien and the neurological signs of Achterberg have great similarity. The triangle could be combined as a basis for the lattice, whereas the square and circle can be viewed in the web. It may be that there are symbols inherent within our consciousness that provide us with guidance, whether they be externally or internally programmed.

Reviewing these categories of symbols and assuming that symbols originate from one or more sources—our neurological makeup, psychodynamics, bodymind association, natural observation, culture, collective unconscious, or as a pure form (prehumankind map)—we see that the power of a symbol is actually derived from the fact that there are multiple layers of meaning for the individual. Without attempting to verify the relationships between the symbol origins, let us explore a theoretical layering of symbols and evaluate how the sources of power in such a system might look:

Origin	*Symbol*		
	Spiral	Mother	Chevrolet
Pure form	X	X	
Collective	X	X	
Culture	X	X	X
Nature	?	X	
Psychodynamic		X	
Bodymind	X	X	
Neurological	X		

While there probably aren't discrete boundaries between the different layers of the symbols involved, it does seem that the symbols that have references to the largest number of sources also have the greatest impact. For example, the symbol of "mother" may have more potential for triggering a process of transformation than does a spiral or a Chevrolet. However, we should also recognize that any symbol can metamorphose, as, for example, a spiral could eventually transform into a snake and the Chevrolet could evolve into a father figure.

Since symbology as a study shows us that a symbol cannot be divorced from the individual experiencing it, the sources of symbols can serve as a framework for understanding and empowering the patient's chosen images. Moreover, the images can be actualized through art, dance, poetry, music, and crafts, so that they can be recognized by and shared with the community. For example, if the patient's imagery includes the adoption of a power animal, such as a turtle, for protection of the self, legends of turtles can be told, shapes of turtles with special meanings can be drawn, turtle songs and dances can be performed.

The community can thus empower the image, often creating a healing symbol for the group.

As in dreams, in imagery there is no definite power base for any given symbol. Instead, like a language, the symbol can serve as a crude condensation of innermost consciousness.

THE SYMBOLIC LANGUAGE OF IMAGERY

Imagery is not so much a "technique" as it is a language in which meanings are imposed upon symbols from a wide variety of influences. It is a complex language expanding from words alone to include auditory, olfactory, visual, and kinesthetic avenues of expression, and it includes the profundity of both ordinary and nonordinary realities. In addition, it includes each individual's total lifetime of experiences and personal semantics. As such, creating this language of imagery is a difficult process that requires patience and careful listening.

In this chapter I have divided the imagery process into parts so that the health care professional can better understand it. But this fragmented analysis should not take the place of listening to the patient with an ear attuned to that person's individualized responses to symbols. For example, a teenaged boy might respond more powerfully to the symbol of the Chevrolet than to mother, since he might richly endow the car with all his hopes and dreams for the future. Whether the images are expressed in song, music, movement, or a story, the power and meaning of the imagery can come from multiple realities. Regardless of the intellectual capacities of the patient, the exact source of an image's power can only be partially understood at a conscious level; the rest is a mystery. The majority of content is stored and shared in the unconscious of all people participating in the process. That is one of the reasons that people in a therapeutic group who have only listened to the described image of another can often have great insights if they can allow the collective unconscious to work for the benefit of that person.

In my experience, the "story" of the physical dimensions of disease, or the metaphor that those dimensions offer from the level of biology, is often the story of a person's life in a larger sense. For example, a woman with severe endometriosis who was also developing adhesions and scar tissue from surgery visualized her body as a fortress with all of its resources being directed into some form of protection. With this image came the awareness that she had learned, as a child, to be feisty and overguarded. Her aggressiveness was a key feature of the way she interacted with others. Her case suggests that it may be possible that the behavior of cells within our bodies can mirror our personalities.

As I have discussed in the book and kit entitled *The Cure*, symbols can be brought into awareness through story and fable with the added dynamics of the hero's intention.[24] Many times the patient can be encouraged to create a story that depicts a path toward wholeness, or at least toward hope. Through whatever means the individual chooses, the hero of the story can manifest the courage and skill to achieve success in the face of the disease.

Intending to use the imagery to effect change is another step beyond simply understanding the symbols. Merely wishing something to change is not enough, and struggling with the "right image" is often a fruitless journey. One can suppose that the image is merely a reflection of the soul's expression, and that its language involves a multiplicity of dimensions—emotional, physical, spiritual, intellectual—that are impossible for us to totally comprehend. However, we do not need to understand it all. To assume that total comprehension of the process is necessary would be a little like saying that we would have to be able to fully comprehend all the processes our bodies go through to digest a hot dog. If that were so, we'd die of old age (and starvation) before we finished eating. Similarly, even though the treatment of choice for the removal of warts is imagery, no one really knows the physiological mechanisms that make it work.

Where getting rid of warts is concerned, nearly anything works for *somebody*, whether it is burying a washrag at the crossroads on a full moon, patting a frog, or massaging the wart with goose oil. No one can tell a person what physiological imagery to use, because no one really knows. Intention itself appears to communicate to the mysterious forces of the body to work in an integrated way for change—in this case, to rid oneself of the wart.

Imagery gives form to our intention but we should remember that the success of our efforts will depend on how clear we are in the process of choosing our symbols. For example, there is a vast difference between changing the kind of car we drive and changing the course of a major disease in our lives. In most cases, the latter requires a total, integrated effort, whereas the former requires changing only a small part of our values and self-image.

Imagery and symbol therapy might not be necessary if the underlying wisdom and intention of our body-mind-spirit were totally known to us. Imagery is our way of exploring and getting a clearer perspective on these deep questions. That is one of the reasons why healing that is accomplished without the patient's taking any responsibility is rarely lasting. For example, bypass heart surgery has been shown to be ineffective for the long term, unless patients also develop a willingness and intent to change their lifestyle and attitudes. Laying on of hands may have some positive effect on a problem, but unless the patient also takes responsibility for changing, so that his or her lifestyle supports health, the problem will recur. Imagery can help us actually understand the processes of change—how to learn from them and integrate them into our lives. Granted, working with healing imagery is a difficult and time-consuming practice, but it provides a bridge to a new place of connectedness and support for the kind of lives we want for ourselves, our loved ones, and our patients. While imagery practice sometimes seems to focus on the symbols of change, it also provides the process—the path toward wholeness and responsible healing.

Interview with Carl Simonton, M.D.
Director of the Simonton Cancer Center
and author of *Getting Well Again* and *The Healing Journey*

Frank Lawlis: Carl, you have been a pioneer in the treatment of cancer from a mind-body point of view for many years. You obviously believe that the mental state has some relevance to the physical state. How did you come to focus on this relationship?

Carl Simonton: Cancer patients—especially the ones who got better—triggered my interest in the connection between the mind and the body. There were very few, if any, psychologists or physicians in the early days who were trying to develop the linkage of how the mind could be used to make us well from cancer.

FL: How would you summarize your current thoughts of how imagery therapy works for the care and management of cancer?

CS: First of all, let me say that imagery is a tool, not the whole protocol for helping a person deal with the dynamics of disease. Yes, I believe that imagery, as a therapy, can be highly effective in helping a person mobilize his or her healing forces for health, but it is one of many effective therapies. Let me say it this way: we know that emotions significantly influence health and recovery from disease in many ways. They are a strong driving force in the immune system, influencing neurotransmitters, hormones, and every component that we know about healing.

We also know that beliefs influence our emotions and, in so doing, influence our health. If you can get people to shift their belief system, it will make a tremendous difference in their emotions and health status. So my point is that imagery is a very powerful tool in terms of addressing the belief system, with the potential for empowering a person to be successful in this sort of approach.

FL: So what you are saying is that there is a deeper source of mind-power than what we call imagery. These would be the belief systems.

CS: What I want to embrace is that the term *imagery* is not merely the visualization of white blood cells and cancer cells in battle, but it can be extended to all realms of experience—family, community, cultural, and spiritual realms.

FL: Can you describe some specific imagery approaches that you are using?

CS: The imagination plays an important role in illness and health. In receiving a disease diagnosis and then participating in a discussion regarding treatment and prognosis, the patient begins to become aware of the doctor's thoughts and emotions, such as hope, fear, dread. The chances are that he or she experiences a combination of images, positive and negative, healthy and unhealthy. And all affect the body at the cellular level.

I use a five-question test to challenge these beliefs and images as to whether they are healthy or unhealthy. Basically the five questions are:

1. Does this belief or image help me protect my life and health?
2. Does it help me enhance my short- and long-term goals?
3. Does it help me resolve or avoid my undesirable conflicts?
4. Does it help me feel the way I want to feel?
5. Is the belief/image based on fact?

If the patient can answer yes to three or more of these questions, I consider the image as relatively healthy. If there are fewer "yes" answers, I encourage the person to shift or challenge these images as healthy.

FL: I have heard many people describe this as "positive thinking." Is that what you would call your approach?

CS: No. Positive thinking is based on the idea that you control your thoughts for only optimistic outcome, and your body will respond accordingly. I think that patients get into trouble with this, especially when it doesn't work at this simplistic level. I prefer to consider my approach "healthy thinking," which takes into consideration the choice and responsibility of the patient. Let's take an example. Consider the three statements:

1. I have cancer, so I am going to die a horrible death.
2. I have cancer, and I will recover fully as long as I think I will.
3. I have cancer, and I have many powerful resources for help. I can make a difference in the outcome and how I feel about it.

The first two statements, a negative thought and a positive thought, ignore the choices of the patient and the process of learning what one's disease and health are all about. They also place a lot of blame on the patient, if things do not go as projected. The third is healthy because it expresses a belief that allows "yes" answers to the five test questions mentioned above, and it promotes an orientation to reality.

FL: So the first two examples leave out the individual's sense of exploration into the meaningfulness of the experience, whereas the "healthy thinking" emphasizes the process of learning and self-examination.

CS: The reason we pay so much attention to beliefs and images in working with patients is that beliefs and images create emotions and, as we know from research and clinical experience, emotions have an important driving force in the components of the immune system. Healthy images increase your sense of power, well-being, and peace of mind. They strengthen your sense of connectedness with your inner wisdom, with others, with the world and universe. Neutral emotions also can be healthy in terms of promoting calmness, peacefulness, but prolonged negative emotions can have unhealthy effects.

FL: I just want to point out that you make a distinction between positive imagery and positive emotions.

CS: Absolutely! Any one image can evoke either a positive or negative emotion, and it is the emotions that are important. For example, one person might image a warm, sandy beach and have peaceful, supportive emotions as a result, but another person may experience fear and anxiety with that image—same image, different emotions. The important lesson here is that if you can change the image, you can control and focus your emotions.

FL: You obviously have a plan for your patients if they are having unhealthy images or beliefs.

CS: The most effective time to work on your beliefs or images is when you are experiencing emotional pain, because then the unhealthy ones are easier to identify. It will be clear that these undesirable emotions are interfering with your life. Here is the process for working on these beliefs and images:

1. Identify the undesirable emotions you are feeling.
2. Take a sheet of paper and draw a line down the middle from top to bottom.
3. In the left-hand column, list five beliefs or images that produce that emotion.
4. Evaluate each image according to the five test questions.
5. For the unhealthy image or beliefs, write out healthier images or beliefs in the right-hand column.
6. Three times a day, in a calm, relaxed state, using your breathing to help you relax, imagine the healthy beliefs. Do this for at least three weeks, until your changed beliefs become unconscious.

FL: An example, please.

CS: Here are some examples of unhealthy images and incompatible healthy ones:

1. I am going to die soon and leave my family regardless of what I do.
   I may or may not die soon, and what I do makes a significant difference.

2. All of my unhealthy beliefs and feelings are making me worse, and I can't change them.
   My unhealthy beliefs and feelings are making me worse, and I can change them.
3. It's doable, but I don't know how.
   It's doable, and I can learn how.

FL: I realize that although we have been discussing imagery, your program is broader than this one aspect. So in closing, perhaps you would want to put imagery in this context.

CS: As I was trying to say in the beginning, imagery is a broad component that is part of many levels of human experience—physical, psychological, and spiritual. The content is applicable to positive or negative emotions. For example, one's imagery of another person can be as toxic to the body as the image of a cancer cell. Interpersonal relationships are very important to our well-being, and these dynamics are addressed in the program.

Cancer is feedback that indicates a need for change—that you need to do more of the things that bring you joy and fulfillment, and fewer of the things that result in emotional pain; that you need to learn to respond to the stresses of life in healthier ways. This message is one of love. Acting on it can help you align yourself with your true nature and significantly influence your body's ability to eliminate the cancer and bring harmony to your overall being.

⫸ 7 ⫷

CO-CONSCIOUSNESS
TRANSFORMATION

THE BEST MEASURE of a ritual's success is that it effects a positive transformation in a person's life. The most auspicious scenario is, of course, when such a change is long-lasting. The person is transformed psychologically, socially, spiritually, and often physically. He or she has a new name, a new role, and perhaps a new way of life.

As an ongoing research project, I collect healing stories. From accounts of patients and participants in workshops both here and abroad, I have by now collected over a thousand stories. I am, of course, interested in these stories because of what they might reveal about the nature of healing, but beyond that I am also interested in exploring their clinical implications. I am also aware of the impact such stories have on others. Patients are always wanting to hear healing stories, as if in search of mythic pathways to be traveled. Success stories encourage them by showing that someone else, possibly very similar to themselves, has achieved a healing. The hope offered by others' stories is especially important when fear and anxiety are clouding a patient's mind, blocking any logical understanding of his or her own problem or its solution.

Brendon O'Reagan and Carol Hirschberg studied "spontaneous remissions" and cures with a slightly different mission in mind—to determine their objective nature.[1] Their conclusions were very similar to mine, though our methods of collecting data were quite different. Two similar elements in particular seemed to stand out: (1) the patients involved had an intent and made an effort to seek a vehicle for change, and (2) they were able to come to terms with a past reality and transform it. Let me explain:

The search for a vehicle of change usually involves a variety of subtle considerations. For example, it is generally true that the probability of achieving a healing is directly proportional to the effort the person invests to find a healing energy and/or healer to work with; what's more, this correlation can be observed in virtually all cultures. One might speculate that there is a deeper element of motivation, expectation, or change of consciousness that becomes involved in this process. We can hardly deny the evidence suggesting that one's commitment to a healing goal actually increases the chance of a positive outcome. This commitment is what we see expressed in those cases where a person sticks tenaciously to a quest for healing.

There is also evidence suggesting that novelty is an important factor for bringing about change and transformation. For example, putting patients in a strange environment, particularly one filled with symbols and situations foreign to them, has a disorienting effect that literally forces them to let go of old belief systems—at least for a period of time—and seek a whole new relationship to the world and the people around them. The element of surprise in which the habitual thinking process of the patient is interrupted can be an important component in introducing an attitude of change. The importance of the physical environment as a special place with unique features, such as a church, temple, or other holy place, cannot be overemphasized. Such an environment takes on a significance of its own as a facilitator of personal change.

The second apparently universal component found in healing stories is a sudden and major "shift" of consciousness, a change of perception that is often dramatic, having a lasting impact on the structure of the personality. This kind of change can be attributed to an altered state of consciousness, but the shift has a deeper influence, ultimately changing a patient's social interactions as well as his or her attentional processes. Metaphors such as "being born again" or "having a spiritual emergence" may describe a major shift of motivation or way of living that can be attributed to a change in the disease status. Friends and family members will note changes in that the patient now responds to situations differently or reorders priorities in his of her life.

For example, Lane was diagnosed with cancer of the pancreas, with a prognosis of approximately two months to live. Although she was only twenty-six years old, she immediately took to her bed and waited for the inevitable decay of her body and mind. However, after two weeks of depression and fear, she began to focus her attention on her twin sons, who were playing in the yard outside her window. As she pondered their future, she thought, "Who is going to raise these children?" Suddenly she was flooded with the sense that she could, and would, be capable of doing so. The message was so strong and powerful that she could no longer take seriously the prognosis of her imminent death.

Lane shifted her self-concept from that of victim, not only of the disease but also in her relationship to her job and her marriage. She began to seek alternative solutions to her disease and a new lifestyle. Recognizing that her old ways of living may have been a factor in her contracting the disease, she decided to "find a new song and dance a new dance."

Lane found several avenues for managing her disease, including imagery, diet, exercise, job change, and a reordering of her life mission. Having been trained as a computer engineer, she shifted to a less technical vocation; she began taking flying lessons and also developed a major interest in mountain climbing. The spontaneous remission of her tumor attested to her success in changing the course of her disease, but a basic shift occurred in all other areas of her life as well.

This kind of far-reaching shift of perspective may be what is required for patients with catastrophic diseases, especially for those with tissue damage. Most of the patients seen at my pain clinics were victims of back injury where trauma and/or surgery had resulted in the growth of scar tissue, which in turn created a major locus of pain. As they would attempt to exercise and stress muscle fibers, the scar tissue, being less elastic than muscle and nerves, created a direct insult upon the structure, resulting in tremendous pain. The scar tissue indirectly acts as a tourniquet that restricts blood circulation, and any increased activity produces ischemic pain for hours. After attempts to exercise and work, these patients are naturally less inclined to want to perform rehabilitation therapies.

After months of restricted movement, scar tissue tends to shorten, creating even more restrictions and pain. Yet without exercise, muscles lose approximately three percent of their strength per day. Consequently, by doing nothing, the patients become weaker and more rigid, with less and less tolerance for pain.

Drugs and surgery are not very helpful in many of these cases. Pain medication often contributes to three new problems. First is the possible inability to recognize physical limits. If persons are so numbed that they can't feel the pain of the stressed tissue, they risk going too far and tearing that tissue, creating more scar tissue as well as delaying healing. Drug dependency is another possible problem; pain medications are psychoactive in nature, with a potential for addiction. In the pain clinics, somewhere between 25 and 40 percent of the patients go through withdrawal symptoms.

A third concern is that pain tolerance may be further reduced. There are long-term effects of pain medications that cannot be ignored. They tend to inhibit naturally occurring biochemicals, called endorphins. As the tolerances for the drugs build, endorphins are reduced, resulting in more sensitivity to less and less pain. We observed that people's tolerance for pain increased by approximately twenty percent merely by eliminating the pain medication.

As one would quickly begin to determine, these pain patients were in a challenging situation. They would have to endure more pain in order to eventually reduce the ongoing chronic pain; they would have to stretch the scar tissue slowly, over many weeks, until there was more flexibility and thus less stress on the nerves and muscle fibers. Scar tissue will stretch, and like a rubber band, if stretched to the limit for a period of time, there will be a gradual release, but the price paid for this desired flexibility is pain. In essence the patient has to experience the hell of spasms and intense aggravation with the hope that there will ultimately come permanent relief. It is not a welcome message for patients, especially as they are just entering the strange and frightening hospital environment.

Yet, sixty to ninety percent of the patients did overcome the pain in exactly the terms described above, and did so with remarkable character. How? I observed that it was impossible to tolerate the horrific pain without shifting to a "co-consciousness," another self that could meet the challenge of transformation. We called upon the patients to bring forth their greater self and strongest inner resources to deal with the struggle. They were asked to give this greater self a name and honor it and to request its help at this time of need. In observing people following these instructions and getting positive results, we became convinced that the process of rehabilitation was one of transformation. To support that process we intentionally and methodically ritualized the embrace of this co-consciousness awareness.

THE MEANING OF CO-CONSCIOUSNESS IN HUMAN EXPERIENCE

The concept of multilevel consciousness was defined as early as 1889 when Pierre Janet postulated that every person has at least two sides to his of her personality, the natures of which might differ considerably.[2] In 1907, Morton Prince suggested that the term *subconscious* might best be understood as the simultaneous activity of two or more systems of awareness in one individual.[3] John Beahrs postulated that we should look upon the sum total of a person's consciousness as the personality.[4]

We might well look to conventional neurological models for help in understanding the source of these multiple levels of human consciousness. In this model, normal consciousness is believed to have its origin in the "triune brain," a hierarchical organization of three mentalities apparently evolving out of the instincts of survival. The oldest component, the *reptilian brain*, includes the brain stem and much of the reticular system. The second level, the *paleomammalian brain*, includes the limbic system and midbrain. The third level, the *neomammalian brain*, or *neocortex*, includes the remainder of the brain components as defined within the neurological model. By virtue of surgical intervention and exacting research into which of our many functions are controlled by which components of the brain, these three components are found to serve us in basic drives for satisfying physical necessities (reptilian), emotions and social interactions (limbic), and intellectual functions and self-awareness (neomammalian).[5]

One researcher postulates that the evolution of human consciousness expanded laterally into large cerebral hemispheres, connected by a bridge of fibers (the *corpus callosum*), which first emerged in the placental animals.[6] With this development, humans achieved the ability to coordinate a rich variety of awareness, ultimately leading to the development of language. The conclusion of this multilevel organization of consciousness is best described by Louis Tinnin: "The human mind is not unitary . . . the sense of mental unity is a universal and obligatory human illusion."[7]

The dominant language area of the left hemisphere of the brain appears to orchestrate the activities of both hemispheres. The language center also takes part in monitoring volition and cognition.[8] However, this monitoring gives a sense of mental unity that is more illusory than real, a fact that is supported by clinical observations and cerebral studies that reveal that other mental systems are competing for recognition even while the person may be experiencing the false sense of unity produced by the language center of the brain.[9] Researchers continue to look for a single unifying center of the human brain, but what they find instead is a complex of motor and sensory functions, such as taste and vision. The location within the body or brain of anything that resembles a unifying *consciousness* continues to elude our best efforts.

Physiologically and psychologically, it is clear that consciousness possesses some means of organizing our attention, and while we cannot exactly pinpoint where that organizing entity is located, we do have a name for it: the governing mental system (GMS). Systems that may have a great impact upon us at any given moment, but that may not be directly expressed in our immediate behavior, are called "latent mental systems" (LMS). Freud's id, ego, and superego represent some of the dynamics of co-consciousness. While the ego serves both the id impulses (reptilian brain) and the superego (emotional or limbic brain), the personality structure is dependent upon a larger overall integrity to maintain itself; the ego does not do it all alone. As long as our egos are healthy and capable of figuring out ways to satisfy our emotional and libidinal impulses while maintaining the awareness of physical reality necessary for our survival, the GMS remains within the egoic structure, with the remaining brain components as LMS. However, if the ego breaks down, we lose the central control of GMS, and psychosis results.

Carl Jung described the features of co-consciousness as "complexes or splinter psyches"; he developed this argument through administering word association tests to patients. He saw the conscious ego as functioning between the external world and the internal, psychic world. Meanwhile he believed that many subpersonalities surround the ego as well, and these might go through many changes throughout the course of our lives. Jung referred to the primary subpersonalities as the *persona*, the *shadow*, the *anima* and *animus*, the archetype of the *spirit*, and the *Self*.[10] He arrived at a hypothesis that divided the unconscious into the personal and the collective unconscious. In this scheme, personal consciousness was seen to contain emotional complexes and the collective unconscious was seen to contain archetypes, that is, "inborn, unlearned tendencies or instincts."[11] One writer summarizes Jung's work in this way: "A complex consists of a cluster of emotionally charged representations. Upon closer examination, one discovers within the complexes a core element that serves as a vehicle for meaning and that functions independently of conscious will."[12] Another explains that complexes and splinter psyches probably develop around an archetypal core. He exemplifies this conclusion by using the "mother" archetype: "The psyche is organized in complexes, each complex forming around and filling out an archetype. The archetype provides the glue that holds the different experiences, inner as well as outer 'mothers' together."[13]

It was probably theorists of the "self" who propagated the idea of a total unity of personality. Using the self for their psychotherapy models, Carl Rogers, Fritz Perls, and others proposed that the basis of human potential, the unity of self, could and should be actualized in all its *potential* capacities. They believed that within a nurturing environment of unconditional love and empathic understanding, the creativity of the self would blossom into fullness. The underlying principle of this model was that in this setting the ideal self and the actual self would come into complete harmony. For forty years, the goals of the human potential movement have been focused on coming to terms with becoming all of what we think we are capable of becoming, of enriching the possibilities of developing a bigger and better self, and of creating a flexible self that could incorporate each aspect of our behavior within one self-structure. In this context, our compassion and kindness toward others are to be combined within the same self-concept as our wickedness and pugnacity. In other words, there is a blending and acceptance of all that we are.

Co-consciousness, Ritual, and Transformation

These models of the self are important to us in that they offer the possibility for transforming our lives and empowering ourselves through discovering a broader picture of what "self" really is. In order to move beyond the obstacles of disease or psychological turmoil, it becomes necessary to *call out* the more appropriate and powerful "selves" at our disposal. For example, it helps to see that we have within us a warrior, a lover, a healer, and a mastermind. It is my belief that ritual is powerful, because it is capable of opening our hearts and minds to these greater possibilities.

Perhaps when we create, through ritual, a new psychic space, the alternative self can emerge and be empowered to take charge of our survival. It is customary to encourage the participants in a power-animal ritual, for example, to dance their animals throughout the night, until they experience themselves becoming what they are in spirit and wisdom. I suspect that this practice is the basis for the were-wolf legends of old, in which shamans literally become their power animals in shape and form.

When we use ritual to temporarily dissolve our everyday consciousness and take on another identity, enormous energy is released. For example, in assuming the character of a wolf, we might let go of guilt that we associate with aggression, passion, and past social transgressions. We are thus free to be focused on the more basic issues of our lives, including sheer survival. In doing so, we perhaps return for a while to having most of our attention focused on the reptilian brain and/or the warrior archtype.

To use a more commonplace example, in rituals designed for the business world, participants are asked to become more creative in either management or product development, whereby *other parts of their minds* are opened. In doing so, they are given the license to express other aspects of their selves; other complexes then come forth and the participants gain wisdom and open up to new directions. One technique is to have people break up into groups of four or five individuals and pretend that they are children, playing games and acting out. Then, the group focuses on how many ways they could use a pencil, or a potato, or some other ordinary object. The people taking part in these "rituals" allow their alternate selves to emerge and conceptualize problems from perspectives they perhaps didn't previously imagine were even possible.

The ability to dissociate from our everyday reality and let ourselves assume other personalities appears to offer numerous benefits for healthy adjustment. By allowing ourselves to "switch over" in this way, we expand our ability to cope with the stresses of everyday life. The following is a brief list of the benefits we may reap from this process:

1. Expanded creativity and ability to blend difficult concepts
2. Mental rehearsal of events or activities
3. Escape from pain and discomfort
4. Integration of the unconscious with the conscious, similar to what happens in dreams
5. Formalization of goals

THE MANY SELVES OF THE HUMAN EXPERIENCE

There are many systems of philosophy and psychology that recognize the existence of subpersonalities, or of our having more than one self. For example, in the system known as transactional analysis, developed by Eric Berne, we see different levels of "ego-states" through which we communicate with other people. Dr. Berne labeled these *parent*, *adult*, and *child*—though it should be noted that the parent and child ego-states could be broken down into more precise complexes.[14]

In his delightful and insightful book *Games People Play*, Berne described different "games," or "transactions," that we set up with other people, depending on which of these three characters we are giving our greatest attention. For example, in the game of "Little Red Riding Hood," the first person begins the transaction in the child ego-state, characterized by frivolous and seductive behavior. The second person assumes a similar child ego-state, and the game begins, looking very much as if the two are playing like children. Suddenly, however, the first person switches character, moving into the parent ego-state, becoming judgmental and imposing a heavy sense of morality upon the interchange between the two. The second person is surprised and confused by the change, which brings up feelings of shame and guilt.

The transactional analysis model sheds much light upon the destructive patterns of certain kinds of interpersonal relationships. At the same time, we recognize that there are appropriate times for each of the ego-states: sometimes we wish to be playful like children; sometimes we need to take a more parental role; and sometimes we need to relate as balanced adults. The implication is that an adult-adult ego-state configuration works best for problem solving; a child-child ego-state configuration might be good when both parties wish to share sexual/ sensual experiences; and an adult-adult ego-state configuration might work best in a situation where two parents need to confront their children's misbehavior. The most potentially troublesome scenarios are when there is a "cross-pattern"; for example, relationships where one person has to be the parent to the other person's child.

In Carl Jung's model, we find a system for looking at masculine and feminine dominant or latent personality types. Building from this system, Robert Moore and Douglas Gillette have described four major masculine archetypes that need to be expressed in a healthy man.[15] Any of the four may be dominant, but awareness of the remaining three is important to understand the true sense of masculinity. The four archetypes are described as the King, Warrior, Magician, and Lover.

The King archetype or complex is characterized by building order and acting out the role of a benevolent father. The Warrior is characterized by loyalty to a higher cause and control over one's own physical and emotional needs. The Magician archetype is one of self-reflection and introspection, looking into the deeper meanings of life. The Lover represents the passionate side of life, someone who has empathy for all of the creatures and energies of the world, male and female.

The implied therapeutic approach of this model is to become aware of and to honor these aspects of being male, to actualize them and integrate them into appropriate life situations without falling into overidentification with any of the archetypes, a common danger. The archetypes are to be used as guidelines but should not be confused as total personality structures. There are excellent opportunities for the King complex to be enacted in contemporary life, with wonderful results; for example, when putting together a new business. However, there are other times that the Lover complex would be more beneficial, as in expressing one's emotional and sensual sides in a romantic relationship, or in listening to the human needs of an employee.

Many of the American Indians had their own personality subtypes. For example, Hyemeyohsts Storm, in *Seven Arrows*, describes four complexes using animal totems: the Buffalo, the Eagle, the Mouse, and the Bear.[16] A person who is a Buffalo would manifest wisdom from an experiential base. The Eagle expresses itself in giving great attention to "the big picture," seeing all realities and giving broad consideration to all problems. The Mouse gives very close attention to details and has the closest relationship with the earth. Being a Bear means using one's gifts of introspection and perceiving life intimately with the heart.

Each animal represents a particular set of perspectives or way of seeing the world. It is generally through a vision quest or through the sage advice of a shaman that a person is asked to consider a change of perspective. For example, a person who habitually views the world as if through the eyes of Eagle may be overlooking details. The "medicine" needed is the perspective of the Mouse, with those eyes we become aware of and attentive to details. As a person learns to shift attention in this way, the shaman may assign new names and clothing apparel as part of a ritual to honor the new personality that is now emerging. The ritual tneds to stablize the shift of perception. For example, the ritual celebrating the shift into adult consciousness from child consciousness—i.e., the initiation into manhood—may help clarify the new roles and responsibilities of the initiate. It is like agreeing to sign a contract that defines the relationship between two or more people.

Multiple Personality Disorder

Within the discussion of subpersonalities and splinter psyches, one must address multiple personality disorder, a diagnostic label that indicates the presence of a pathology. In order to appreciate the basic definition of multiple personality disorder as a psychopathological process, we must consider it as an aspect of dissociation, which has been an interchangeable term with altered states of consciousness (ASC). By dissociating oneself from a normal state of consciousness, one can enter into other realms of being and can discover different selves.

Dissociation, in relationship to multiple personality discovery, was noted by some of the earliest psychological researchers such as Pierre Janet. However, William James's research in the area probably had the greatest impact on the psychological community, particularly among Americans. James stated, for example, that "the mind seems to embrace a confederation of psychic entities."[17]

The pathological components of dissociation appear to be based on three criteria: a major alteration of the sense of identity, the amnesia of events or behaviors in alter-selves, and the traumatic associations involved in the development of the individual coping mechanisms.

Frank Putnam has articulated the pathological process by which a normal process evoles into a disorder.[18] He defines these processes as "state-change" disorders in which a dysregulation occurs in transition between states. In essence, personality trait transition is normal and often required as one changes from one situation to another; however, if the coping, through some traumatic crisis, creates a malfunction in this switch process, one will suffer from the lack of adaptation mechanisms for meeting emotional challenges. If the individual cannot shift to a more appropriate complex, he or she may be neurotically fixed to a specific mode of behavior, even in inappropriate circumstances.

The research on multiple personality disorder has some interesting implications for our potential to bring about physical change through imagery and self-concept modification. For some reason, the multiple personality syndrome has a close correlation to rapid healing. There is also the phenomenon of correlated physical states within the same body; for example, within the same person, one personality may be allergic to a substance while another is not. One personality within the same person may have high blood pressure or arthritis while another does not. One will have skin rashes while the other does not. One may be near-sighted, the other normal-sighted. Would it not be reasonable to assume that similar physical changes accompany psychological complex changes in those not afflicted with multiple personality disorder?

Interestingly, there is a consistent alter-personality reported in most multiple personality cases, called the Internal Self-Helper, known as the ISH.[19] One researcher labeled this entity the "hidden observer," having observed this phenomenon in his experiments with automatic writing and talking.[20] This personality is the entity that resembles the "higher self," in that it has been described as occurring within the person but connecting him or her with a higher source above or outside the person. The ISH is a guide and source of information about what is going on within the personality system; at the same time, it may function as a consultant on the direction the therapy needs to take. Many therapists actively use the ISH for integrating the person with multiple personality disorder.

If multiple personality disorder is merely an extreme form of a normal state in which one can switch to more appropriate personality behaviors, then consideration of the ISH complex within each of us has direct implications, especially within the medical realm. If we can communicate with this entity about our health issues, we will discover a great resource for achieving and maintaining optimal health.

CO-CONSCIOUSNESS AS A RESOURCE FOR HEALTH

One of the major differences between our transpersonal approaches to health and those of the more traditional modes of medicine and psychology is in how to determine what course to take toward the treatment of a problem. Traditionally, we are taught to first determine what is *wrong* with the patient and then correct the problem. In the context of co-consciousness, the approach would be to determine what complex would be *right* with the person; then we would call upon that entity within the patient that has the greatest power and wisdom for approaching that person's health problem. We might especially look for an archetype that might be residing within that person's unconscious. The intuitive decision about which complexes or conscious entities might be available and effective for that individual would be dependent on the experience and sensitivity of the patient and/or therapist.

For instance, in my clinical experience, calling forth Robert Bly's "Iron John" has been extremely important for many men who had felt an absence of this complex, and thus had not been able to exercise their own internal gifts and strengths. Brooke Brown found that for many women the discovery of a "bag lady" archetype within themselves was profoundly empowering.[21] I have found that if a patient can discover a complex or co-consciousness that is appropriate for his or her apparent needs, there is a sense of great empowerment. Their lives often transform from dull routine into an exciting adventure when this occurs.

The arena of superhealth—sports—is full of stories about recruiting personality complexes to deal with physical and mental issues. Consistently the superathletes describe the experience of surrendering their wills to a greater power, whereupon another self takes over and fulfills far greater achievements than they would have done with their more restricted egos. Utah State University basketball star Wayne Estes, who in his senior year ranked just above Princeton's Bill Bradley and just below leading scorer Rick Barry of the University of Miami, scored forty-eight points in his final game. He said in a radio interview, "I was just putting the ball up. . . . Somebody else was putting it in for me."[22]

In the 1953 World Series, George Shuba was the second player ever to pinch-hit a home run in a Series. Blinded by the sun, he could barely see the ball, but afterwards he said, ". . . it wasn't me. There was something else guiding the bat. I couldn't see the ball, and you can think what you want, but another hand was guiding my bat."[23]

My favorite sports story is about Bob Beamon, the world record holder for the broad jump. At the Mexico City Olympics, Beamon was little known for his past accomplishments as a world athlete. Few people, himself included, had any great expectations for him that day. Yet before his jump, he felt a strange calm and a sense of unlimited possibility. As he began his run toward the pit, something else took control. He soared two feet farther than anyone else had ever jumped—an extraordinary achievement—yet he was not aware of his accomplishment until he had moved to the center of the field and donned his warm-up pants. When he was told what he'd done, he became so disoriented that he got sick to his stomach.[24]

Receiving a medical diagnosis of life-threatening disease or a prognosis requiring a major change in one's career or lifestyle, a patient struggles with primal fears and anxieties about change and survival. The stress of dealing with a major threat to one's very existence or self-concept can rock the foundation of one's being. In attempting to cope with one's dominant personality, one may become stuck in a cycle of ruminations about self or begin expressing a mixture of latent complexes such as becoming dependent like an infant, withdrawing from life, or expressing oneself with outbursts of anger.

When patients finally reached one of the clinics with which I was affiliated, they were often in the depths of despression and terribly fearful of the medical system. Whether the person I observed was acting in the dominant complex or had regressed to one of the latent complexes, the typical pattern was fear and anger, with a childlike response to the health care system. I could understand the reaction. After all, the medical care system is confusing enough for an insider, but to an outsider, it is chaos, filled with incomprehensible languages and equipment that is anything but comforting by its presence. The sterility of the atmosphere and the pain incurred as part of medical procedures would be problematic enough, but the authoritarian ambience often triggers a fight-or-flight response.

The personality pattern of acquiescence to authority may not be appropriate when proactive decisions and actions are to be taken in dealing with disease. One of the problems in medical realms is the need for people with severe disease such as cancer or diabetes to take responsibility for their own health. In order to develop the best scenario for their health care, they must be willing to learn about their bodies, to be sensitive to their physical and emotional needs, and to be willing to administer to their needs. In short, they must become masters of their fate. If they cannot shift to this state of mind but instead become increasingly dependent upon others for their care, the outcome is usually poor.

As a first step, we acknowledged what was happening with the patient and focused attention on "healing" the fear and acquiescence syndrome. We also taught the patients and their families about those complexes that they were themselves manifesting. We often did this through stories that illustrated in an accessible, nonthreatening way what they were going through. We also found that it was effective to guide them individually or as a group through vision quests within their own minds, and by having supportive meetings with the therapeutic community. In these ways we were able to explore and discover what aspects of the self, the latent personality complexes, might be available to deal more constructively with very difficult situations.

Although we often made use of the archetypal and subpersonality typologies mentioned previously, they were not applicable to everyone. My approach has been to introduce the concepts of totems and guides, which may come to a patient in dreams or in an altered state of consciousness. After I teach the practices of deep relaxation (through drumming, breathing, etc.) and of maintaining a memory of the journey through drawing or writing, we discuss the need to deal with the problem within a specific frame of mind or attitude. As the patient assumes that attitude, it is expressed in some ritualized form (such as painting a symbol, establishing a name, singing a song, or the like) with the support of the group that we have previously established.

Name-changing has proved to be a powerful approach for maintaining the complex changes that are sometimes involved, using name tags and dress as reminders to the rest of the staff. Implied in a name is the empowered element, as well as the individualized path. For example, we have had "Great Bull Tom," "Swift Deer Janet," "Soaring Eagle Frank," along with thousands of others.

We've consistently found certain personality traits that predict successful rehabilitation through efforts of the kind we describe here. These include what might be termed "cognitive flexibility," the ability to entertain new and unusual ideas and experiences. Whether in the rehabilitation of cancer patients or patients with chronic pain, the most significant predictive measure of success is the ability to change ideas about one's perception of the world or oneself. It would be logical that this would embrace the ability to switch to modes of coping that might previously have been quite outside a patient's realm of experience.

CONCLUSION

In this chapter, we have discussed co-consciousness—enlisting latent personality structures in order to deal with threatening situations. The process is quite complicated. One has to contend with fear and resentment, the resistance to change itself, and the adjustment to the disease. However, what is so magical when we are able to achieve these changes is that they happen naturally whenever the patient gives them a chance. Patients appear to want to discover a part of themselves that has courage and integrity in the face of the problems facing them. It has been fascinating to work with seemingly frail women who have magnificently powerful bears within them, and macho males who have dancers and singers within them. After a while one can feel and see the virtually limitless resources and powerful allies that lie hidden within each of us, just waiting to be called forth. No wonder the shaman laughs when we see ourselves only as a single unified self, unable to understand the depth of ancestral support and spiritual strength the universe offers us.

Traveling to the world of spirits to diagnose and treat illness was a common practice in ancient cultures. Perhaps the point of this art was to bring forth the most appropriate soul or spirit from within the patient; perhaps the disease itself was motivating the unconscious to conjure up the personality needed to address a particular life issue. For example, I have known many individuals who felt blessed by their illnesses because they brought forth their courage and an attitude necessary for dealing with long-standing vocational or relationship issues as well.

Co-conscious shifts are critical events in transformation and transcendence. Unless there is a major change into a more powerful consciousness, the individual simply does not have the capacity to change. This stands to reason since the present personality complex could indeed be responsible for the state of health or disease in which the person finds him- or herself. Through ritual, we can become aware of a greater power than the self, empowering extraordinary selves to come forth to help the patient in his or her healing or other efforts to become more whole. This ability is an extraordinary gift, requiring great skill to embrace, but it is a uniquely human opportunity.

‖≡‖

Interview with James Fadiman, PH.D.

Author of *Health for the Whole Person*
and *Personality and Development*

Frank Lawlis: What is the difference between multiple personality disorder and the kind of multiple consciousness that you discuss?

James Fadiman: First, I want to say that I feel that modern psychology and psychiatry have been mistaken in treating multiple personality as a disorder, rather than regarding people with this condition as not having handled their multiplicity well and having become dysfunctional as a result. Multiple personality is connected to every other part of the mental apparatus; it is not this small part out to the side. What I have observed is that the psychiatric community likes to treat everyone who is a clear multiple as if it were a disorder because they are threatened by the existence of multiple selves. There is not a high level of acceptance for physicians with another view, because there is such a desperate hold on the theory of the single self.

I prefer to distinguish healthy multiplicity from pathological multiplicity. Pathological multiplicity is where there is not a shared memory among personalities, which leads to breakdowns.

FL: From your definition, the absence of shared memory is the pathological aspect of the whole issue?

JF: It seems to be. We should also discuss the phenomenon of splitting a piece off from the rest of the experience. When part of you is paralyzed with fear or pain, and another part of you is able to flee and get away, that is what you do to survive. In extreme situations, the human mind dissociates in order to survive. We see this in the enormous amount of literature about child abuse and also in the literature about war experience. The war literature talks about adult behavior; when you interview these people, they understand completely that dissociation is normal and lifesaving in war. Afterward, some veterans have inappropriately repressed memories and show disorders, but most of these people can be helped to work out these memory disorders without being labeled multiples.

FL: How would this data relate to our models of psychotherapy?

JF: The new model would be that you would not insist on a totally consistent behavior in all situations, which would be an expression of only one aspect of the self. The model would insist upon the "right mind at the right time," which is to have access to the personality traits that would be appropriate to the situation, accompanied by an appropriate skill set. The model would recognize that different sets of skills accompany different personality sets, even in the pathological studies. The most interesting example of this is the different personality dynamics one sees when people are bilingual. My research with bilingual therapists has shown that they are all sensitive to the shifts in their personalities when they switch languages. They are aware that their emotions change and that they think about things differently.

FL: Do you think that the ability to have multiplicity of consciousness is inherent in our genetic structure, or do we learn how to do it?

JF: I think that we learn how to add on to the skills that are required by our environment. For example, in the case of these bilingual people, they have some experience in adapting to a new set of circumstances under good conditions. I suspect that the soldier who has developed the ability to split from his experience will always have that ability. On the other hand, those people who have been raised in a very gentle and restricted way may have a less developed ability to split, and may have less access to themselves. So when we refer to the term *provincial*, we may be referring to a person who has less ability to adapt well to different environments. Whereas the term *cosmopolitan* may relate to a person with a wide range of adjustment skills. When we look back in their lives, we find that they have a lot of experience in shifting personalities.

FL: Is experience the emerging modality of consciousness?

JF: Yes. For instance, every kindergarten student can learn to play a musical instrument. But by the sixth grade, the percentage of children who can learn has decreased. It is a normal predisposition to play a musical instrument, but it is the experience that allows that predisposition to develop.

FL: I have used the example of calling forth the "warrior" to deal with disease. Is this something that is consistent with your model of mental health?

JF: It is most exciting to me that there is some part in us that is good at healing. One of the reasons is that we can then put one person to work on healing full-time. If we are using imagery techniques, we know that fifteen minutes twice a day is good, but if there is a consciousness with a focus on it six hours a day, that's even better. One part of the personality can be working diligently while other parts can be handling the outside world. That may be a plausible reason why multiples have such outstanding recuperative powers. Schizophrenics, also, are some of the healthiest people we know of.

In the training programs that evoke the "healer" and can give the healer skills, and then give the healer space to accomplish its activities without restraints, healing occurs very well. I think that is the way of the medicine of the future.

FL: Is there a common thread in all the complexes in a multiple personality, such as intelligence or temperament?

JF: The biographies that I have read, mainly about people who are pretty disturbed, say no. There are differences in sex, IQ, artistic abilities, age, and others. There are skill sets: one complex can be a fine artist and another can barely draw a simple figure. So it looks like the pressures that make for a large skill set come from a very wide range of experience. The desire for an underlying connecting identity or skill set is a holdover from the one-self theory.

There is an argument currently going on in the *Journal of Humanistic Psychology* around whether or not there must be a conductor of the orchestra, meaning an overall master or coordinator of the personality.

It might be reassuring to think that there is, but my picture is more of the rotating leadership that you might see in a flock of flying birds. There is no leader for long, because such leadership has a fatigue factor. In fact, it may create the neurosis that we see in depression and anxiety. A more adaptive way is to have a rotation type leadership within the personality.

FL: So in your paradigm, the "hidden healer" would not be in charge at all times, either.

JF: Yes, which is also true with the inner destroyer. It seems that each of us also has personalities with destructive potential, such as smoking or overeating. These complexes simply do not understand that these behaviors are not healthy. One of the ways you work with them is to get them to participate in the effect of the destructiveness, rather than going out and getting drunk and allowing another part to take the guilt and hangover. The hidden healer is usually accessible to most of us, but its voice is easily overwhelmed, probably because our culture does not support it nearly as well as the destructive complexes. If you ask any smoker if the habit is good for them, none will say yes. But if you ask them to stop, they will reply that the process would be impossible or the pleasure is too great. If you ask the hidden healer about the habit, it will reply that it is not in control of the body when the habit is being indulged.

FL: Do you bring the hidden healer into your therapy?

JF: I might bring in the "designated driver," the complex in charge that has the appropriate skills for the problem. Sometimes the hidden observer is not the best one to work with. It may be a quiet part that has special skills in learning or in dealing with someone else. It is always a little dangerous to begin to assign courses of action too quickly.

One might also access "higher level" beings who seem to be more helpful and more wise, but have less control. They usually consider themselves not as part of the body, but only passing through to help the person. At this point the multiplicity theory gets a little ragged, a little confusing. But if you ask people in a light trance state if there is a part that would be helpful, there is almost always a positive response.

Some of these entities may not be a permanent part of the self. They may be more like angels than psychological dynamics. These experiences are different from "channeling," but I am not clear at this time how they fit into our model.

Our theory of a separate self is not held by other cultures. In India, you are living with many uncles and aunts, and you have a dream. It is not assumed that that dream belongs to you. It is part of the family, and can be claimed by other members of the family as their dream. When I research children who live in a group constellation for long periods of their lives, I find that their identities become massed in the whole community. As with twins, imagery and self-identity becomes a different concept from that of personal space.

FL: What is the definition of psychological health?

JF: There are two parts: the ability to bring forth the most appropriate entity for a given situation, and to have harmony. The goal of therapy is not unity, but harmony, similar to the harmony present among physical aspects of the healthy body. Each organ has its own function, but a healthy body is in harmony with all of its parts. From a psychological perspective, in a harmonious person, each voice is distinct and separate, yet the blend is one that is created by the mixture of voices. It is like a well-organized football team, in which each player has its own reason and function, but they are all going in the same direction.

⫸ III ⫷
SPECIAL ISSUES

⁙ 8 ⁙

DEATH AND
TRANSITION

I N THIS BOOK WE have been discussing transpersonal modes for
dealing with transition and transformation. Death is the ultimate
transition. Throughout the ages, spiritual traditions have stressed the
importance of dealing with the death experience. Exposure to rituals
and other transpersonal therapies has always played a positive and effective role in preparation for death. They can even have self-tran-
scending and life-transforming qualities for people who are not dying.

Yet death in our culture is a process to be denied, even disdained.
The medical community and public health organizations consider it an
enemy to be defeated. For health care professionals, death is the symbol of failure and incompetence. As a society, we have denied the existence of death, hoping for science to eventually save us from this
ultimate embarrassment. In the meantime, we often fail to acknowledge the necessity of learning to cope competently with this reality,
losing the opportunity to empower ourselves to face life's major transition.

As transpersonal health care professionals, we can recognize certain fundamental fears and tasks inherent in the dying process and help the patient work with them through ritual, counseling, and imagery. Embracing the inevitability of death is a prerequisite for personal evolution, and, in truth, it is death that makes evolution possible.

In preparation for death, a person becomes highly aware of the ultimate inevitability of loss of self-identity and release from the reality to which he or she is now oriented. There is no longer any need to fortify a persona, and the urgency to finish "past business" presses him on toward the utmost honesty. In working with terminal cancer patients, I have had the privilege of dealing with a variety of individual processes. What all have had in common is purity of motivation and genuine expression of feeling. In many ways the interpersonal transactions with such individuals are similar to the intimate responses one finds in sexual relationships. There is a closeness and loss of boundaries in a caring and loving atmosphere. There is also a fairly uniform spectrum of issues that arise for individuals who are dying.

Fears of Death and Transformation

The greatest obstacle in transition is fear. Based on clinical experience as well as research, six basic fears are associated with death: fear of the unknown, fear of suffering, fear of loneliness, fear of interruption of life plans, concern about the impact of one's death on others, and the fear of nonbeing. There are predictable psychological coping methods involved in facing these fears—denial, anger, depression, negotiation, and acceptance, for example. No matter what the coping mechanism, the magnitude of the transition that death entails continually challenges the individual toward deeper and deeper levels of transformation. The anxieties only represent obstacles to the natural evolution of consciousness.

1. *Fear of the unknown.* In some sense, at the root of all the anxieties about death is fear of the unknown. One of the primary functions of religions is to present a view of an afterlife so that one can have some sense of what to expect after death. It becomes a clear possibility for those who believe in a hell that everlasting torture may await them. There may also be the expectation of some judgment process, rather

like the "final exam" of life. Whether these mythologies came into being as a way to take the edge off the fear of the unknown, as an incentive related to the need to "finish business," or as propaganda with the motivation to make people follow a particular moral code, they can engender dread and guilt in people with a terminal disease. It is of utmost importance to acknowledge these feelings and listen to them with care.

2. *Fear of suffering.* Anxieties about the potential pain and suffering of dying are expressed by many people with terminal disease. An underlying fear is that one will be humiliated. The thought of being violated by an unbeatable force makes people feel victimized, assaulted. The prospect of becoming increasingly helpless engenders depression and anger in many individuals. The thought of losing control of one's bowels or having to be fed is embarrassing and shameful. Therefore, loss of pride is also a major issue.

People also fear suffering the loss of power, loss of control that we strive throughout our lives to maintain. Faced with ultimate surrender to invisible and incomprehensible forces, the dying person also fears the psychological suffering that the loss of self might entail.

3. *Fear of loneliness.* The process of death is lonely. There is literally no one alive who has had the complete experience and lived to tell about it. The dying person is often shunned, as if death itself were contagious, even if the disease is not. Others do not know what to say to him or her, and they may be afraid of being asked an embarrassing question, such as "Am I dying?" Hospitals have made the process even more isolating with strict visiting hours and restrictions that limit visitors to family members. Moreover, even with the most loving support, the dying person is faced with the realization that ultimately he or she will make the journey alone.

4. *Fear of interruption of life plans.* Many individuals in the last stages of disease feel that they are dying "before their time," before being able to accomplish their goals, and they experience a sense of disappointment and failure. When my father was on his deathbed, he remarked, "What really upsets me is being put on the bench when I want to be in the game."

5. *Fear of the impact on others.* People worry about what will happen

to their families and loved ones after they die. Their concerns may center around financial or emotional support, or simply around the impact that their absence will have. The dying person may also be concerned about providing a good role model in dealing with the process. One man said, "I just do not want my son to see me weak and unable to take care of myself. It will frighten him. I must be strong to the end."

6. *Fear of nonbeing.* The ultimate fear of the ego is to cease to exist, and most of us spend our whole lives protecting and defending it. It is very difficult to face its ultimate dissolution, or the fact that perhaps it never really existed in the first place. The illusion of solidity leads one to project a brittle interpretation of matter and events and is a major obstacle to opening and surrendering to the dying process. As Stephen Levine elaborates in his book *Who Dies?*: "The more we have invested in protecting something of 'me,' the more we have to lose and the less we open to a deeper perception of what dies, of what really exists. The more we hide or posture or postpone life, the more we fear death."[1]

As people attempt to cope with the frightening aspects of life change, they often go into denial and anger, two destructive methods for coping. Relaxation techniques are excellent for coping with fear, especially in grasping the reality of the death cycle. If individuals can enter into a state of release, they can lower their resistance to change, which allows them then to explore greater dimensions of self, of life, and of the natural evolution of consciousness. I have consistently observed persons reaching some acceptance of the idea of change and indeed the necessity of change to allow a broad experience. We may have to release some of those things that we held as precious, but there are also things that we may *want* to release, such as a sick body, a demanding lifestyle, a relationship, even a financial debt. There is no blame or punishment, only the correct season for change.

THE TASKS OF TRANSFORMATION

As we begin to confront the reality of transformation through death, there are three tasks to be accomplished: release of expectations for the future, release of the past, and recognition of what is and what is not the self. As major shifts in consciousness occur, there is a natural tendency to regress into passivity and self-absorption, perhaps because of fear or the novelty of the experience. What is helpful at this stage is actively to release our concepts and fixed ideas about reality, so that we can approach the transformation in an open, accepting state. Holding on to our ideas of how things are or should be can hinder the process of transformation in significant ways. In some sense, what these three tasks point to is the value of living in the present moment.

1. *Releasing expectations for the future.* We plan our future around goals and live our lives in an attempt to accomplish them. Many of these goals may be unconscious. There is, for example, normally a drive toward power. Whether we are aware of it or not, we often act to promote our superiority over others and define ourselves by our abilities, success, and accomplishments. Our self-concept and self-esteem can become entirely dependent on past successes and future realization of our goals. Each accomplishment serves to strengthen our self-concept, and the greater the goal, the greater the self-concept might be. Many people with whom I have worked have become totally tied to the future, merely tolerating the present. "When my ship comes in . . ." is an expression that articulates perfectly this psychological expectation of how much better life will be when the future finally arrives.

Impending death has the tendency to bring things very much into the present. The abrupt interruption of future projections when there *is* no foreseeable future can throw the self-concept of individuals into chaos, especially if they have depended upon future goals as integral to their sense of self. It can be very challenging for such people to be forced suddenly to live in the present and retain their self-esteem. The person's feeling of not being grounded can bring out further competitiveness and aggression as he or she tries desperately to grasp something "solid."

In my work with individuals, I often address release in two stages: *holding on* to life in hopes that the ultimate fate and transition will be avoided, and *letting go* of the control long enough to allow for the bereavement that must take place.

Out of fear of the unknown, we often invest a lot of energy in denial of inevitable change, regardless of how good or bad we may perceive it, in order to keep things in some kind of order we understand. I find it difficult and even problematic to rush this phase. Because of the enormous amount of energy consumed in this particular psychological defense, the denial will usually play itself out in a fairly brief period of time. It is important for those engaged in helping during this period to be patient, supportive, empathetic, and caring, while waiting for the point at which the "holding on" will resolve and a more integrated perspective can be approached.

As the "holding on" is released, the "letting go" begins to take place. At this stage, we can give the patient the space, time, and support needed to say goodbye to his or her future hopes and expectations. These are losses to be grieved and disappointments to be shared. A listening ear and silence are usually enough to be helpful, but sometimes it is useful to ritualize the end of dreams and visions so that the patient's ambitions and expectations can be turned over to another or released altogether. In one instance, I was with an individual who had dreamed of inventing a toothbrush that would always be clean. As the family and I held his vision, he concluded the ritual by saying that he would take this project to heaven with him. In some way he had made peace with his apparent lack of fulfillment.

2. *Releasing the past.* There are two aspects to releasing the past: forgiving and grieving. Dying people need to make peace with individuals who hold significance for them, and it is important that unresolved emotions such as guilt, self-criticism, resentment, blame, and depression be aired. To forgive is to release the imprisoned consciousness from the past. Not forgiving creates an obstacle to the open state necessary for transformation.

Forgiveness is also essential to cultivating wholeness and healing in ourselves and others. The process brings the total sense of the self into the present, freeing the negativity attached to past events. As Stephen Levine writes in *Healing into Life and Death:* "In the deepest stages of forgiveness, one finds that there is no 'other' to send forgiveness toward, but just a 'sense of being' shared. The one mind, the one heart in which we all float. Then, as unconditional love, there is not forgiveness for another, but forgiveness with another."[2]

Individuals can be encouraged to act out in reality visualized experiences such as approaching an old friend or parent to express love and gratitude for past events. Sometimes the imagery of forgiveness for someone who is no longer alive is sufficient to release imprisoned feelings.

Although it is clearly important to forgive others, a more critical issue for transformation is to forgive oneself. Self-blame is a major obstacle to receiving love and support from others and allowing oneself to surrender in trust to the grace of the universe. Unless we forgive the part of ourselves that we deny, we will continue to suffer the pain of punishing ourselves for not being perfect.

Grieving over what we are losing is a natural stage of release. For this reason, it is important that the grief be supported and not denied. The purpose of grief counseling is not to help us forget what we are losing or have lost, but to help us adapt to the loss. With patience and the proper processing, ultimately the loss will be transformed into meaningfulness.

3. *Asking, "Who am I?"* Delving into the question of what is self and what is not self is a very practical approach that can help clarify relationship issues. We typically perceive the world through a veil of beliefs and concepts, reinforced by language. As we face death, the more we hang on to the concepts and beliefs about "me," the more we experience hope and fear, which increases suffering.

It is interesting that in most rituals, one of the prerequisites is surrendering one's name, which is replaced by another one during the ritual. This represents surrendering our self-concept on a very basic level. The interesting question then arises, "If I am not my self-concept, who am I?" What part of the self survives death, what part dissolves?

I find that this process is the most interesting part of counseling. Through it may arise the realization that an individual is more than his or her productivity, more than the role of a father or mother, more than the labels we stick to ourselves. We often go through a ritual of imagining our own funerals, listening to what our friends and family say about us and thinking about what our lives meant. As we review our experiences, relationships, and values, we become aware that we have been on a mission guided by our particular personal vision all of our lives. The ultimate answer to the question "Who am I?" can easily be resolved in positive terms.

Throughout this book, we have presented findings that the *transpersonal* aspect of human experience is not bound by time and space. Relaxing into that larger realm of consciousness through imagery, an altered state of consciousness, or some form of meditation can help the dying person begin to let go of his or her limited self-concept and begin to identify with the larger view.

WHAT WE CAN LEARN FROM NEAR-DEATH EXPERIENCES

As we confront death, we are moving into unknown terrain. There are no "authorities" on the afterlife. Yet there is plenty of relevant information from those who have had near-death experiences (NDEs) about what passing the threshold of death entails. Raymond Moody has identified the following core components of an NDE: ineffability, hearing news of one's death, feelings of peace, a buzzing noise, a dark tunnel, awareness of being out of one's body, meeting deceased loved ones, the being of light, the life review, and the frontier.[3] Based on his study of 102 individuals who had lived through NDEs, Kenneth Ring has described five phases of the process: an intimation of death preceded by the overwhelming feeling of peace and calmness, the observation of the soul and body separating, the transition into another reality (often traveling through space or a tunnel), the awareness of a brilliant golden light, and becoming one with the universe.[4]

Obviously each account of an NDE bears its own personal and unique stamp; however, the general consensus is that the process is almost always positive. According to Ring's studies, the aftermath of an NDE almost always involves a positive change in one's self-concept.

Based on his own near-death experience and the literature of NDEs, August Reader, M.D., has identified the five psychological phases of dying: fear, release, sense of peacefulness, the perception of light, and contact with other entities with the choice of return.[5] With each phase, he has also traced the physiological process of the brain's response. Interestingly enough, his findings imply that we have physiological mechanisms that "hardwire" us into the experience described by people who have gone to the threshold of death and returned.

With the awareness of death comes intense fear and stress, taxing the sympathetic nervous system to its maximum. As Reader points out, the body has a built-in mechanism to modulate the fear response to the process of death by resetting the cardiac function to a slower pace, thus allowing our consciousness to respond automatically to the challenge with a sense of peace. Thus, approaching death is often a peaceful experience rather than a frightening one. In other words, the body and mind attempt to adapt to the stress by putting their functions in balance, which creates the feeling of release and surrender.

Then, as the brain begins to attempt to conserve oxygen for its most necessary functions, the temporal lobe is stimulated, which enhances imagery. This catalyzes a review of all life experiences that might help one out of this physiologically dire situation. This review may include information from genetic or transpersonal sources—in other words, it may include instinctive as well as experiential knowledge.

The blood supply is directed to the occipital lobes, stimulating a white light or tunnel imagery, so common also in migraine headache victims. This physiological explanation may help in understanding the reports of people who have experienced near-death. Perhaps we are all "hardwired" via the neurological pathways in preparation for this transition.

The exciting conclusion one draws from Dr. Reader's observations is that there seems to be some physiological mechanism that opens the individual to transpersonal realms at the time of death. His research also shows how we are able to access wisdom beyond the ego boundaries at some point in the process. What is really intriguing about this process is that, as the research of Moody and Ring shows, the ultimate outcome of an NDE is consistently a focus on altruistic motivation, which may have a physiological basis. Considering this outcome, it is interesting to note that many initiation rituals for spiritual movements include a practice such as baptism (drowning) that would bring one to an NDE, and that the initiates are then referred to as "reborn" into a new way of thought and behavior. Such rituals have long been popular in the Celtic and Native American cultures. Another interesting point is that Buddha, Jesus, and others went through near-death experiences before becoming spiritual teachers.

TRANSITION ENHANCEMENT

NDE is not a terminal state, but a process of transpersonal shift in perspective, from inner focus to altruistic motivation. Some of the effects of NDEs can be replicated through other transpersonal processes such as peak experiences, ASCs, rituals, and extreme illness, which parallel the death/rebirth process and can help us prepare for that ultimate transition. Aging and maturation—any process that takes us beyond our childlike behaviors and self-concepts—is also helpful practice for facing death.

As we have learned more about being helpful to others who are dying, what we have discovered from the work of shamans is that practice is useful in preparing for the experience. The transformational cycle is natural, and not every transformation ends in physical death. As we have already seen, ritual involves surrendering the self and giving up previous attachments, which is a kind of death. Therefore guided rituals can be very helpful to the dying person by "rehearsing" the journey in the company of a fellow traveler.

Similarly, imagery rehearsals also help the dying person deal with the impending transition. Many exercises are designed to help the patient experience death at an imaginal level. Relaxation and coping imagery also have been very helpful in dealing with the management of pain and discomfort on a physical level and with the issue of suffering on a psychological level.

The process of dying can only be addressed in the transpersonal realm, since none of us really knows what the ultimate experience is beyond our personal conscious reality in this life. As John Schneider has pointed out, resources from that higher realm—wisdom, joy, unconditional love, surrender of selfish motivation and intention, openness, and energy transformation—are readily available to both the dying and those left to grieve.[6] And it may require very little effort or formality to tap into that realm. In counseling the dying, I have learned that one readily available entryway into the transpersonal realm is simply to listen to the patients' stories. I have always been surprised at how much I learn if I let my curiosity be the guide, and also at how much benefit I can be to others by listening. I have heard stories of unsolved murders and love affairs, of intense suffering and hostilities, and of lives hardened by the inability to forgive self and others. My experience has taught me that the human spirit is immortally powerful and courageous.

As the patient and I come to trust each other through this process, we go into altered states of consciousness almost automatically. I do not need to guide the imagery, merely to structure it so that the wisdom beyond our rational egos can come into our reality. These quests are always calming to the patients as well as positive in their messages.

Is the transitional process through life stages, especially death, generalized and preset neurologically or is the process different from person to person, psychologically or spiritually? From my review of the literature and clinical observations, I have concluded that both statements are true. From a psychological perspective, dying individuals display a variety of human characteristics and meet the challenges of death the way they have met other life changes—adolescence, aging or trauma, and other developmental stages. If a person has great fear of change, then that person will have great fear of dying. The same defenses and abilities will be employed as before.

In counseling the dying, it is helpful to know what their previous coping style has been so that one knows what to expect. Even qualities that might be seen as shortcomings can be redirected into strengths. For example, many people habitually engage in power struggles, using anger and aggression against the object of challenge. This could potentially be quite destructive for the self. However, if the energy of the power struggle can be refocused and channeled into a warriorlike approach to death, it brings honor to the process instead of shame.

Just as each person's dying process is marked by his or her unique psychological and physical attributes, so there are universal aspects of the experience, perhaps spurred by spiritual or neurological processes. My own observation, which is in accord with the available literature, is that if the fear can be resolved, dying is a positive experience, even among children. There appears to be a prescribed path through the doorway of existence, whether preordained by the culture or by personal experience.

Through my experience as a clinician interested in transpersonal medicine, I can attest to the value of the "psychopomp," one who serves as a guide in such transitions. My knowledge of altered states of consciousness, imagery, and alternate realities has served me well in understanding and supporting the wonderful patients who have shared their deaths with me. This experience perhaps most accentuates the difference between a psychologist and a shaman: whereas the psychologist focuses on the rational coping mechanisms of consciousness, the shaman shares and even redirects perceptions of reality and self into a space beyond rational mind. If one can open to the transpersonal realm and step to the threshold of the unknown as the patient releases his or her hold on the physical state of being, the experience can be shared as holy and perfect.

||≡|||

Interview with John Schneider, PH.D.

Professor, Department of Psychiatry, Michigan State University,
and author of *Stress, Loss, and Grief*

Frank Lawlis: What interventions do you practice during the death and dying process?

John Schneider: I try to relate to loss and grief as a transformative process. One of the important things is to connect the process of dying with other transformative events throughout the life of the patient. It is upsetting to people to see death as a unique experience, a foreign and unpredictable experience for which they have no preparation. I try to show them that their other life experiences can help them understand the process of dying, can help them get in touch with it as an extension of many other transitions in their lives. We discuss how they have dealt with change before, and who they were in the past in contrast to the present. Much of the fear of death is the fear of the future. We do not know the future, but then we did not know the future ten years ago either. People get some reassurance out of tying the death experience into a consistent pattern of life. When they can relate it to a natural pattern connected with their other experiences, it is not so foreign, alien.

FL: When you work with people, you apparently focus on the death experience as another developmental stage?

JS: I approach a person as a life story, as the story of a life process instead of a death event. I help people see death as a part of their whole life story, their personal myth. How does it fit with their history? Does

173

it have meaning to them in context with other things they have dealt with?

I remember working with one terminally ill man who was very depressed. He was mute, and everyone was attempting to help him adjust to his condition. It was difficult at best. The one thing he could relate to was how much he used to enjoy fishing. As I asked him his experiences, he began to use physical expressions to demonstrate some of his joy and excitement. Out of remembering his passion for fishing, he began to deal with his condition and how he was going to cope. It took his going back to a piece of his life that was very important to him. Fishing was really a metaphor for his whole life.

FL: Are you saying that hearing someone's "life story" or personal myth is really the first step in helping them in transformation?

JS: Yes. It is ironic that so many people are in settings in which no one really knows their life stories. I think that the essence of why people feel so dehumanized in the dying process is that there is no one there to hear the life story.

So having someone hear your life story is an important step. Incompleteness is a real fear; dying people have a need to finish the story. Part of this need may be the need to pass on the myth, which might have a life of its own, and in any case needs to be received and appreciated in some way. And whatever the last chapter is has to be included. Part of the depression that many people feel at this last stage of their lives is that no one is really interested in it, especially in hearing the ending. The family can be so caught up in the emotion—"Oh my God, this can't be the last chapter! Maybe if I don't listen to it, it won't happen"—that they can't relate to the person's need to tell the story, to experience a sense of closure before death comes.

FL: Most of us have an idea of what a "good death" would be, but what is a "bad death"?

JS: I have two perspectives on "good" death and "bad" death. First, what does the death leave for the survivors? A "bad" death can leave them with an enormous fear of the transformative experience itself. It might also leave them with a sense of incompleteness about the relationship. My father died very suddenly when I was eighteen. I really don't know what the experience was like for him, but I knew that he had been very depressed some months before he died because a dream he had had apparently dissolved. What I got from his death was the message "Don't dream." If you dreamed and your dream did not come true, death was the immediate result. It could literally kill you.

The other aspect of a "bad" death concerns the individual who is dying. When the patient resists the process, there is increased suffering and pain. Dwelling on the issues of unfinished business, on things that we did not get to do, tarnishes our personal myth because we feel despair at "giving up." Instead of surrender, there is a sense of failure. The whole sense of timing is confusing.

Yet one never really knows when one will die. The person with a terminal illness who actually has time to experience the different stages of release is in a luxurious situation. In a sudden death, there is no time to prepare. This awareness can help us live each day to its fullest potential, as if there were no tomorrow. Each day could have a completeness in itself. I think this is really what we should be talking about in trying to define a "good" death. Opening to transformative experiences is opening to the full experience at any time. Whatever it takes for us to arrive at this conscious opening is important. My father's death certainly was a major part of that realization for me. Don't hang on to anger or unforgiveness. Deal with it on the spot, because you may otherwise never have the chance to completely deal with it.

FL: So you see life as a gift to be appreciated every day?

JS: In grief we understand what we may have lost, and at the same time we come to appreciate what we have received as gifts. What we lost could diminish us, but it also could increase our capacities to live more fully. The gift of life, regardless of how long it is ours, is a cause for celebration.

Have you heard of the "Iris principle"? The Greek goddess Iris was the goddess of suffering. It was her role to help people let go of what was already gone, because holding onto things that were no longer there causes suffering. Iris had to do with forgiveness, lost love, lost dreams, attachments in general. For example, she would clip a lock of a dead person's hair and release them from life. So often we maintain the illusion that what is truly gone still exists in its identical form. We have a hard time fathoming impermanence, even though it is around us all the time. For example, a lot of young people really believe that they will live forever, if they play their cards right.

FL: Do you base your work on the phases that Elisabeth Kübler-Ross has identified in the death process?

JS: The phases Kübler-Ross identified are really more involved with the process of struggling against the death, rather than the process of transition. I think that you have identified the transformative issues much more completely than she has. Her system is too simplistic for me in that regard. There need to be some therapeutic aspects to the process, and that involves the recognition of transition in meaningful ways.

FL: Is a belief in life beyond the physical boundary necessary to help patients through the dying process?

JS: Belief in an afterlife of some sort is an essential aspect of approaching death positively. It is very positive to see something beyond, just as, in grieving, it is essential to see that there is something beyond our ego. There is more to us than this physical presence. If people cannot believe that, death will be a frightening experience. This is not necessarily a religious belief, but a basic instinct that there is something more than this skin sack we call our "selves"—a broader consciousness, a relationship dimension, or other constructs that we define generally as transpersonal. Even atheists can accept that. The people I observe as having the greatest difficulties are the people who have not decided what they believe yet. They have a real dilemma, to decide what is there for them after death.

⦚⦚ 9 ⦚⦚

HUMOR AND
TRANSFORMATION

I N AUGUST 1964, Norman Cousins, editor of the *Saturday Review*, was diagnosed with ankylosing spondylitis, a severe disintegration of the connective tissue in and around the spinal column. This disease causes extreme pain throughout the body, with a very small probability of recovery (one chance in five hundred). The sedimentation rate—the speed with which red blood cells settle in a test tube measured in millimeters per hour—is used to measure the progression of the disease in terms of the level of inflammation in the body. Any measurement above 40 is considered significant disease process. As Cousins's rate soared above 115, pain and paralysis quickly overwhelmed him. His doctors were at a loss for effective treatment.

As an experiment in self-treatment, Cousins began watching humorous films, listening to humorous talks, imagining himself healthy, and taking large dosages of vitamin C. His sedimentation rate began to fall. By the end of the eighth day of this unorthodox "treatment," he was able to move his thumbs without pain, and the gravelly nodules on his back and hands were receding. Although it took quite some time,

Cousins fully recovered from his disease, becoming a leading advocate of alternative medical approaches.

Through the popularity of his book *Anatomy of an Illness*, Cousins's story has become one of the most famous having to do with recovering health through humor, but it is not unique.[1] Philosophers, psychologists, and physicians have studied humor for its medicinal effects. Plato and Aristotle considered laughter an adaptation response,[2] and Darwin researched laughter as a stress resolution feature peculiar to the Homo sapiens group.[3] Freud pondered over the use of humor in psychotherapy in a paper titled "Jokes and Their Relation to the Unconscious."[4] Gordon Allport,[5] Abraham Maslow,[6] and Carl Rogers[7] have each acknowledged humor as a major attribute of healthy personalities.

Some years ago I met with Pete Conchos, spiritual leader of the Taos Pueblo. When I asked him what ingredients go into the healing process, he answered, "Forgiveness and laughter." He then explained that if we do not forgive one another, our souls are captured in a time trap in the past. Laughter helps break us out of that particular prison and allows us to move forward.

Forgiveness has been recognized as a primary therapeutic activity in all of the programs with which I have been affiliated and with all of the patients with whom I have worked. The power of humor has also greatly impressed me with its transformative potential. When patients are asked what components of their programs were the most significant in their recovery, group support and humor are frequent responses: "Once I begin to laugh, my pain starts to recede and I can see life from a different perspective."

In investigating humor's capacity to change people—how it works, and how it could be applied—my literature search revealed only that by the time the behavior, the psychological theories, and the neurological linkages are examined, scientists' analyses of qualities related to humor resemble the postmortem of a rat. Many have evaluated the muscular reactions of the smile response, associating it with the social and psychological environment. Others have studied the reactions of the abdominal muscles used in laughter and correlated them with biochemical changes in oxygen increases or decreases in the brain. Mathematical equations of humor have even been developed: [$C =$

f(TrCLx)E], where *C* is the cure or outcome, *T* is the therapist, *CL* is the client, *r* is the relationship, and *x* is whatever we might refer to as "humorous."

As for so many processes that elude logical understanding, the only definition of humor that begins to be comprehensive is a deductive one: humor is the mechanism that causes laughter or mirth. And yet, such a definition does not begin to describe the dynamics of humor in the transformative process, where it is a powerful tool among methods for transcending pain and suffering. As such, it has a history of effective use by healers and therapists.

HUMOR AS A TRANSPERSONAL PRINCIPLE

Michael Harner, author of *The Way of the Shaman*, once said to be wary of anyone claiming to be a shaman who did not have a sense of humor.[8] A real shaman sees many dimensions of reality at once and is constantly amused by the ironies and paradoxes they present. He or she knows that life is never what it seems. We have seen the transpersonal principle of multiple realities demonstrated in our discussions of the multiple layers of the personality complex, altered states of consciousness, and the nonlinearity of time and space.

Humor shifts one's awareness of realities, and we meet the sudden change in perspective with laughter. Although, on the surface, humor may be incongruous with any given situation, the shift often reduces tension in trying to solve whatever problem the situation presents. The change of orientation or interruption of linear logic can reorder the energetic field or response to a broader perceptual field, offering new problem-solving strategies or a shift in attitude. Even the language and emotions we use in approaching the problem may change. Neurological patterns and physiological transmissions are changed by laughter; a healthier response to a situation can result.

Humor can evoke a childlike authenticity and a simplification of values, which can be helpful in conflict resolution. For example, the need to "win" an argument or debate may be dissipated as both parties see the humor in their disagreement. That in itself creates a new plane of understanding, reducing fear of loss of self-esteem.

ELEMENTS OF HUMOR

The essence of humor is that it is unexpected and embodies an element of surprise that startles us out of our habitual frame of mind. In his films, Charlie Chaplin physically incarnates this element of surprise. In one scene, the villain is chasing the heroine down the street. The camera cuts back and forth between the fall guy and a banana peel on the sidewalk. At the last second, the heavy sees the banana peel and jumps over it, landing in an open manhole.

There are three elements of humor that are related to this shift in consciousness—*status shift, incongruity or ambivalence,* and *release.* Humor equalizes the status of people when it targets a group of people whose social standing may be intimidating, such as doctors and politicians, because it brings them down to the status of the listener or observer. It serves as an assurance to the insecure that everyone is human and makes mistakes. Examples:

> Artificial hearts are nothing new. Politicians have had them for years. (*Mack McGinnis*)

> Supreme Court Justice Sandra Day O'Connor went with the other justices to a restaurant for lunch. The waiter asked for her order first. "I'll have a steak sandwich and coffee." "What about the vegetables?" asked the waiter. O'Connor said, "Oh, they'll have the same."

Humor can also introduce incongruity and ambivalence into a seemingly solid situation by bringing two or more contrasting realities into one thought. It couples a component of ordinary reality that everyone preceives with some aspect that should not coexist. By focusing on the absurdity of a situation or exaggerating it, we see its funny side. In a dishonest world, even honesty is amusing. Examples:

> If you think the world makes sense, then how come hot dogs come in packages of ten and hot dog buns come in packages of eight? (*Robert Wohl*)

We shouldn't criticize potholes. They're among the few things left on the road that are still being made in the USA. (*Robert Orben*)

Humor provides release, which helps reduce tension or frustration, especially when the target of the joke is relevant to the point of conflict. Often the psychological dynamic is related to embarrassment or the loss of self-esteem. Even when we drop a glass of water or someone points out an innocent error we made—much less when we are ill and may feel embarrassed by it—we laugh and make a joke of our inadequacies. Release reduces stress. Examples:

I learned about sex the hard way—from books! (*Emo Phillips*)

I finally had an orgasm, but my doctor said it was the wrong kind. (*Woody Allen*)

I've got all the money I'll ever need—if I die by four o'clock this afternoon. (*Henny Youngman*)

THE STRUCTURE OF HUMOR

In cartoons and skits, jokes and stories, the four basic structures for jokes are *double entendres*, *reverses*, *triples*, and *paired elements*. A *double entendre* uses an ambiguous word or phrase to change the reality of the story.

Secretary to boss: "I've got good news and bad news. The good news is that your wife is keeping a cat around the house, so she won't be lonely when you travel. The bad news is that the cat's six-foot-two and plays jazz clarinet."

The most common form of the double entendre format uses a pronoun that means a hundred different things, like *it*.

Examples:

> Lawyers do it in their briefs.
> Doctors do it with patience.
> Bankers do it with interest.
> Elevator operators do it going up and down.

The literal meaning of a key word used in this way makes linear logic illogical, forcing the reader into almost childlike comprehension. It can also be seen clearly in stories about what children say. For example:

> Grandma Jeanne was babysitting, and every five minutes four-year-old Brianne made another request to avoid having to go to sleep. Exasperated, Jeanne said, "Brianne, if you call Grandma Jeanne one more time, I'm going to get very angry." Five minutes later she heard a quiet little voice: "Mrs. Lawlis, can I have a glass of water?"

The *cliché*—an extension of the double entendre—takes a familiar way of thinking and gives it a twist. Examples:

> Every twelve and a half seconds, some woman in the U.S. is giving birth. We've got to find that woman and stop her.

> Q: Why was George Washington buried at Mount Vernon?
> A: Because he was dead!

Rather than using a play on words, as in the double entendre, the *reverse* shifts the ending of a story so that the listener has to consider another cognitive framework to conclude the picture. An example:

> One day I was playing—I was about seven years old—and I saw the cellar door open just a crack. Now my folks had always warned me, "Whatever you do, don't go near the cellar door." But I had to see what was on the other side if it killed me, so I

went to the cellar door, pushed it and walked through, and I saw strange, wonderful things, things I had never seen before, like trees, grass, flowers, the sun. That was nice. (*Emo Phillips*)

They just took away the license of one of our doctors for having sex with his patients. And that's too bad, because he was the best veterinarian in town.

Triples are the most common structure for jokes. This structure is based on the preparation, the anticipation, and the payoff. Here is an example:

Waitress (with a hoarse voice): (preparation) "For dessert, we've got ice cream—vanilla, chocolate, and strawberry." (anticipation) Customer: "Do you have laryngitis?" Waitress: "No, just vanilla, chocolate, and strawberry." (payoff)

Is Humor Therapeutic?

Various efforts have been made to show that humor is therapeutic; however, few results appear to be capable of determining its effect across methodologies. One study investigated the effect of counselor-introduced humor on client discomfort and found some support for the effect of humor when compared with a waiting-control group (which has been put on a wait list and is used as a control group without treatment) and an attention-control group (which is given forms of attention other than the experimental condition and is used as a comparison group).[9] However, another study found that humor did not have a significant impact on tension or anxiety-change scores of the clients.[10] The results of another study showed that the participants actually preferred therapists who did not use humor in dealing with their problems.[11]

One researcher tested the effect of exposure to comedy on human participants to determine changes in brain activity. In a series of experiments using instructed hyperventilation and different kinds of comedy, he was able to conclude that the people who responded to the comedy did have higher concordant EEG readings compared with those who did not, and that the humor had a more powerful effect than the instructed breathing pattern.[12]

Results of another study suggest that a good belly laugh can prompt the brain to block manufacture of immune suppressors such as cortisone or speed up production of immune enhancers such as beta-endorphins. This study found that laughter increases the heart rate, blood pressure, breathing rate, and blood oxygen, followed by reductions frequently below normal levels.[13]

Another researcher concluded that laughter increases breathing activity and oxygen exchange, increases muscular activity and heart rate, and stimulates the cardiovascular system, the sympathetic nervous system, and the production of catecholamines like epinephrine, all of which stimulate the production of endorphins, the body's natural pain-reducing enzymes.[14]

David McClelland of Boston University compared the immunity measure of secretory immunoglobulin A (S-IgA) in the saliva of students who were shown films of W. C. Fields and Mother Teresa. Temporary elevations (one hour) were noted in the comedy film, and there were also increases measured for the participants' responses to the film about Mother Teresa.[15] A university study used a similar method by showing episodes of *Candid Camera* with other film and relaxation tapes, using the dependent variables of changes in mood and skin temperature, skin conductivity, and heart rate. It concluded that the humorous film was effective in reducing stress, although students had a range of different responses.[16]

The mood-elevating effect of laughter is assumed to be based on a biochemical mechanism involving various neurotransmitters. When we laugh, an inhibition of depression occurs; hence, a norepinephrine elevation results in a seratoninergic involvement. Norepinephrine is a hormone that is related to high-stress states and the serotonergic process is a neurological interaction among a variety of brain functions that features a neurological coping mechanism for stress and anxiety. The involvement of catecholamines has been demonstrated by the use of the anti-Parkinson's drug levodopa into the reduce pathological laughter and may indicate an organic human need to laugh as a compensation mechanism.

The most provocative results of the studies have been short-term stress-lowering physiological changes. This would suggest at least that humor opens the door to shifting the physical and mental status quo. However, in spite of the experience of Norman Cousins, it would be difficult to assume—based on the prevailing research—that humor alone can cure disease.

APPLICATIONS OF HUMOR
IN TRANSPERSONAL MEDICINE

Humor can be a valuable assessment or therapeutic tool. A patient's favorite joke may provide helpful clues to the underlying process of his or her personal path. Humor can be used to alleviate tension, overcome resistances, rethink solutions, respond more appropriately to a situation, and form healthier relationships with the community. It may even open a door to previously disavowed experiences, making it possible to confront repressed emotions. Certainly, humor can help broaden communication.

Although many have cautioned against the use of humor in psychotherapy, psychologists from Freud forward attest to its role in the reduction of suffering. The literature points to fourteen basic contributions of humor, at least in functional methods for conducting the process of therapy. These are:

Clarifies self-defeating behavior
Provides means to explore new solutions to problems
Relieves monotony of ongoing problem-solving
Shifts overseriousness of therapy process
Interrupts paradoxical or irrational thinking
Reduces grandiosity
Reduces helplessness
Enhances interpersonal relationships
Reduces anxiety, stress, and tension
Redirects or reduces hostility and aggression

Increases ability to reframe situations
Facilitates the learning process
Provides a diagnostic aid to underlying needs
Demonstrates therapist as competent
Enhances therapeutic alliance
Helps break through resistance
Helps self-observation
Provides an outlet for hostile feelings
Provides a new form of communication
Provides free-association material
Helps confront "sacred cows"

Applying a humorous perspective is an art. It requires judicious choice of subject, words, timing, depth, and method of delivery. Humor can be used as a direct or indirect weapon, in repartee or word play, to provoke, challenge, get attention, probe, defend, and relieve tension. It is an important way to teach, vent emotion, reinforce self-esteem, seduce, tease, share thoughts, express joy, truth, and creativity. With humor, we can transcend ordinary reality. It is a natural function of "having fun."

Like any tool for transformation, humor is a two-edged sword. While it can create opportunities for the patient, it can also serve in detrimental ways. Without sensitivity to the emotional state of the patient, the therapist using humor can unconsciously make the patient feel ridiculed, lowering his or her self-confidence. Humor can also be a thin mask over hostility or aggression.

Almost any day-to-day situation offers an opportunity for the health care provider to introduce humorous reality-shifts pertinent to a patient's concerns. For example, in order to diffuse a patient's anxiety, I have told stories about what has happened to me in my own anxious moments. Gentle teasing, exaggeration, and self-criticism are also excellent ways to help create rapport with a patient. Shifting one's own perceptions of a reality that feels very solid can help lighten up a situation. I often tell a joke on myself to dispel a sense of separateness between myself and another individual, which can be especially helpful in a hospital situation when one is wearing what can be an intimidating white coat. For example:

> One night, years ago when I was flying my own airplane, my son Tiff was accompanying me to a professional meeting. We ran into a snowstorm, and I was very uncomfortable with the situation, but since Tiff had a weak stomach for flying anyway, I pretended not to be concerned about the weather. We finally reached our destination after a very rough and complicated route. As we rested in the airport, Tiff asked, "Dad, were you nervous?"
>
> I quickly replied, "No, I am an experienced pilot. We learn to deal with weather like this all the time."
>
> He continued his inquiry, "Are you nervous now?"
>
> Again, I replied in a confident manner, "No, I am just thinking about the meeting tomorrow."
>
> To which Tiff replied, "Then what are we doing in the women's restroom?"

As elsewhere, in the clinical setting humor can be accidental or planned. However, it is hard to program humor. Its very nature is rooted in surprise. In the clinical setting, the sudden shift in reality may be confusing, and the patient may misunderstand the health care worker's efforts. Sensitivity and intelligence are crucial to using humor toward constructive ends.

The situations that present an opportunity for "accidental" humor are blessings. One example that comes to mind concerns a time when we were experiencing some racial tension in one of the pain clinics. The patients included four blacks, two Hispanics, and six whites. One of the white men was very prejudiced and outspoken, which created a definite sense of unease in the group.

One day I was demonstrating the therapeutic use of massage for stress and pain management, with instructions for breathing and relaxation. I was working on one of the black women. When I put some mild pressure on her back, she farted. Silence prevailed for what seemed to be a very long time, but then she began to laugh. I hugged her and laughed along. The prejudiced man soon joined us, saying, "We are all human." Soon, the whole group was laughing and shouting, "We are all human, after all." That became a group slogan and the group became a community.

The shift from experiencing separateness to connectedness was complete. It was a healing and forgiving experience that did not particularly have to be talked about, although it represented a major step for everyone. I could not have planned it. It was a gift of opportunity.

In fact, I rarely plan humor in my interractions with patients, although I do have some standard interventions that help shift attitude. As one would suspect, most of the chronic pain patients who have come to the clinics are angry—angry at their families for not understanding them, at their doctors for not fixing them, at their employers for hurting them, and at themselves for feeling useless and unproductive. Profane language is common in expressing their feelings and descriptions of various personnel. Sometimes I lead a discussion of profanity usage in which I go for the most offensive phrase in the group experience. Without exception, the term is the phrase "Fuck you."

I always prepare the group by requesting permission to discuss profane language, to utter some words as a means of teaching how we articulate our emotional response to pain. I facetiously explain that I believe that the word *fuck* was derived from the legal term for the charge brought against people who are arrested for performing illegal sexual acts: For Unlawful Carnal Knowledge. Then I talk about how I personally have only pleasurable associations with the act of sexual intercourse, the thought of the act, and my partner in the act. I consider being told "Fuck you" a blessing. If anyone tells me, "Fuck you," my response will be, "Thank you very much." This evokes laughter and opens a new relationship with me based on language that uses old terms in a new way. I have shared my humanity with the community and opened the door to a new reality.

Like many other forms of art, humor has lost its connection to its original purpose—to transform. By introducing it as a major component of transpersonal healing, using it consciously for individual, community, and global needs, perhaps we can begin to institute its broader application in the field of health.

Interview with Larry Dossey, M.D.

Author of *Space, Time, and Medicine; Beyond Illness;* and *Healing Words*

Frank Lawlis: What does humor have to do with the transpersonal realm?

Larry Dossey: When we laugh and play, we have some of our most vivid experiences of nonlocal reality. As Zen scholar and translator R. H. Blythe put it,

> Laughter is a state of being here and also everywhere, an infinite and timeless expansion of one's nevertheless inalienable being. When we laugh we are free of all the oppression of our personality, or that of others, and even of God, who is indeed laughed away.[17]

FL: Do you think humor has lost some of its power as a transformative form in our Western culture?

LD: Life, we have said in Western culture, is grim. As a result of our serious outlook, play, laughter, and humor have taken a beating. But even within the West there has been a constant stream of insight that the humorless life leaves out something vital. For example, Goethe wrote, "The man of understanding finds everything laughable; the man of reason, almost nothing." Schiller: "Man is only human when he is at play," and Schopenhauer: ". . . a sense of humor is the only divine quality of man."

A life that has no humor or play is one in which insecurity, fear, defensiveness, rigidity, and fanaticism have an advantage. These are all aspects of a local, limited sense of self, a personal ego that defines itself only in terms of limited space and time. The more hypertrophied it becomes, the more it shields one from apprehending a nonlocal sense of reality. With time, life seems "dead serious"—contracted, distorted, walled-off.

FL: Do other traditions seem to value humor more?

LD: Many traditions have described the relationship between laughter and seeing the world nonlocally, as it really is. The Indian sage Ramana Maharshi (1890–1950) said:

> There is no greater mystery than this—that being the reality we seek to gain reality. We think there is something hiding our reality and that it must be destroyed before the reality is gained. It is ridiculous. A day will dawn when you will yourself laugh at your past efforts. That which will be the day you laugh is also here and now.[18]

An Apache myth relates that the creator made man able to do everything—talk, run, look, and hear. But he was not satisfied until man could do just one thing more—laugh. And so man laughed and laughed and laughed. Then the creator said, "Now you are fit to live."[19]

FL: How does humor relate to other transpersonal experiences, such as meditation?

LD: Humor and meditation accomplish some of the same aims. Both help us let things float away; they show us that we are not the center of the universe; they allow us to open to our nonlocal, transpersonal universe.

Closely related to laughter and play are experiences of enormous happiness—those moments that are genuinely rapturous, exalted, ecstatic. One of the literal meanings of the word ecstasy is "standing apart." This definition is instructive because genuinely ecstatic experiences involve a feeling of nonlocality, of standing apart from the here-and-now. As one escapes the world of local experience—the limiting, constricting sense of the ego and the self—one may enter into a boundless, unconfined domain of pure experience.

⁗ 10 ⁗

PAIN AS A
DOORWAY TO
HEALING

P AIN COULD BE DESCRIBED as an experience of physical or psychological suffering that brings the patient to the threshold of the
possibility of transformation. Pain becomes destructive when it solidi-
fies a concept of punishment or shame; then the person in pain falls
into the inescapable self-concept of being a victim and is unable to
change. Cultural imagery and constructs, secondary gains that may be
realized from "victimhood," and psychological trauma may all contrib-
ute to such a solidification. At the root of such self-limitation is a lack
of understanding of the transpersonal dimensions available to both the
patient and the health care worker. If patients can lean into their pain
and experience it fully, they can educate themselves in the subtleties of
the experience and how it affects their self-image. This is the beginning of success in pain management. However, the greater point is that
truly experiencing and working with pain allows patients to undergo a
transformation that may open them to new possibilities for contribution to the community and even the culture at large.

PAIN IS RELATIVE

In our culture, pain is considered "bad," something to be feared, avoided, denied, and repressed. We seek pleasure to avoid pain. Yet pain is relative. We can see this by looking at rituals that illustrate different perceptions of the reality of painful stimuli. For example, in parts of India the hook-hanging ritual is still practiced, in which someone is chosen to channel the power of the gods into blessing the children and the harvest.[1] Nonsterilized steel hooks are shoved under the chosen person's skin and back lumbar muscles. The hooks are attached to strong ropes that are used to hoist the man up, bringing his full weight against the hooks in his back. Throughout the two weeks he hangs there, he shows no sign of distress or discomfort. Afterward, there is no sign of infection or scar tissue. Similarly, in the Sun Dance ceremonies of the North American Plains Indians, two skewers are pushed under the skin of the breasts of young men and attached to a pole by a rope. In this ritual, participants eventually tear themselves from the skewers, again with no sign of pain or infection.[2]

The relativity of pain can also be observed by looking at cultural differences in the experience of childbirth. Anthropologists have long noted that throughout the world there are cultures in which women demonstrate no distress or pain during childbirth.[3] Interestingly enough, in some of these cultures the fathers appear to experience the pain in place of the mothers, even to the point of requiring convalescence for their ordeal.

Outside the context of ritual and childbirth, further cultural differences in the perception of pain have been observed. For example, in laboratory studies levels of radiant heat are reported as "painful" by people of Mediterranean origin, while those of Northern European descent describe them simply as "warm."[4] Other studies have demonstrated that women of Italian descent tolerate electric shock more easily and with less pain than women of Native American or Jewish origin.[5]

The perception of pain can also vary according to the situation. One study compared soldiers' requests for morphine to those of civilians with similar surgical wounds and found that the civilians claimed much greater pain and demanded pain-relieving substances more frequently. The conclusion drawn was as follows:

> The common belief that wounds are inevitably associated with pain, and that the more extensive the wound the worse the pain, was not supported by observations made as carefully as possible in the combat zone. . . . The data state in numerical terms what is known to all thoughtful clinical observers: there is no simple direct relationship between the wound *per se* and the pain experienced. The pain is in very large part determined by other factors, and of great importance here is the significance of the wound. . . . In the wounded soldier [the response to injury] was relief, thankfulness at his escape alive from the battlefield, even euphoria; to the civilian, his major surgery was a depressing, calamitous event.[6]

As the research has focused on the qualitative aspects of pain, an important concept has developed regarding the cognitive complexity of the experience. In essence, the term *cognitive complexity* describes the multiple dimensions in which a person can construe his or her feelings, life events, and the world in meaningful terms. It seems that the simpler a person's imagery of the pain experience, the less capable the individual is of understanding subtle issues of the experience, thereby making it more stressful. For example, if pain, whether it be physical or psychological, is perceived in global dimensions, solutions are also global and not particularly applicable on a personal level. On the other hand, the more complex or vivid the description of the pain, the more meaningful the experience can be when integrated with other life events.

For example, following up a study by Jeanne Achterberg, Linda Kenner, Kris Kopetz, and myself, which compared the pain imagery of blacks, whites, and Mexican-American chronic back patients,[7] Mitch Murry measured the cognitive complexities of the pain images of these three groups.[8] He found that the degree of pain responses and stress response was directly related to lack of cognitive complexity. The results demonstrated that having a complex understanding of the experience of pain, as well as a variety of ways to describe it, was very helpful. Less cognitive complexity reduced the ability to understand the subtle aspects of pain and was related to greater depression and less positive progression in the pain-management program. The narrower the concept of the pain image, the more difficult the pain management. The group with the most simple terminology, the Mexican-Americans, had the greatest difficulties and greatest stress, which was predictable because of their language barrier. (However, I would like to interject a word of caution in terms of stereotyping people of different cultures. Differences between individuals are always greater than those between people grouped by cultural background, especially in regard to dealing with catastrophic events.)

The emotional context of the pain experience also significantly affects how it is perceived. For example, a research study of a group of Bariba (a major ethnic group inhabiting northern Benin and Nigeria, West Africa) found that self-inflicted and socially inflicted pain, especially through rituals such as circumcision and clitoridectomy, were considered courageous and honorable; the participants did not describe them as painful. However, other kinds of pain—particularly those inflicted as punishment—carried with them an emotional construct of shame. These were described as extremely painful.[9]

How to Evaluate Pain

We have used two methods to effectively evaluate a patient's capacity to shift his or her perception of pain. Both offer some degree of sophistication, at least in their ability to clearly predict why patients relate to their chronic pain as they do and what expectations one might formulate in regard to their response to a pain-management program. While other evaluation protocols are available, in my experience with patients from a variety of cultural backgrounds, these specific approaches have been the most useful.

The Image Pain Drawing Technique invites expression on a nonverbal level and thereby minimizes the language barrier.[10] The patient merely draws the image of the pain on the profile of a human figure, using personal or displayed symbols to denote the sensations and intensities of the pain pattern. For example, if the patient feels pins and needles down her back and through her right leg, the image of pain could be expressed by small straight lines in the back and right leg of the figure. Often patients draw unrequested features, such as axes and pitchforks, which have explanatory psychological value. The simplest scoring scheme for this evaluation is objectified by counting the number of grids within the human body profile.[11]

Combined with the scoring system and the visual analog intensity scale, the Image Pain Drawing Technique appears to have the highest reliability in terms of understanding at least the level of intensity of pain across individuals and time. It helps the clinician assess the degree of relief supplied by surgery, drugs, counseling, or any other intervention used. We have extended the use of the Image Pain Drawing Technique to include some implication of cognitive complexity using a scale of 0–100 to delineate subtle differences in the pain, which helps the patient and the physician see qualitative progress in management of the pain.

This assessment technique also allows the patient to use actual words or mental concepts to qualify the pain that can give the clinician insight into the emotional construct from which the experience is perceived. For example, words like *bad, burning,* and *biting* imply pain as a form of punishment. This inquiry into how the patient associates the pain emotionally can clarify the cultural as well as the personal aspects of the painful experience.

The second instrument found remarkably predictive of success in rehabilitation programs and constant across many cultures, including Argentina and Japan, is the Health Attribution Test.[12] This questionnaire, which takes only ten minutes to complete, purports to measure the attribution or cause of general health. In essence it asks the question: "Why do I have pain and what will make me well?" By addressing these issues, it reveals the basic personal medical model of the individual, that is, the belief system to which he attributes health or illness. Using a formatted scoring feature, this method can produce a profile in minutes that shows whether the patient attributes his health—or lack of it—to internal resources, powerful others, or fate.

Patients who score high on internal resources see their health as a matter of personal choice and responsibility. As might be expected, these patients do very well in any kind of rehabilitation program (pain clinic, cancer rehabilitation, vocational rehabilitation, and others). The second factor relates to how much value one places upon others (including God) for good health, from total dependence on them to simply depending on them for advice. High scores can connote dependency (which can enhance inpatient success at times), while low scores can connote a stubborn resistance to changing lifestyles (a common score among physicians). Those with high scores in the third factor—fate—are very poor candidates for a rehabilitation program because they lack any belief system that will enable them to project an image of success.

TRANSPERSONAL APPROACHES

There are many philosophies and program organization plans for pain rehabilitation programs, ranging from the Fordyce model of high-intensive behavioral modification to the social learning model to cognitive relearning models. In the context of addressing pain management that has societal and cultural overtones, the primary focus of intervention consistent with successful rehabilitation is the modification of the pain experience. There are currently three primary transpersonal approaches for altering the perception of pain: relaxation therapies, control techniques, and meaningfulness counseling.

1. *Relaxation therapies.* Relaxation therapies cover a wide variety of techniques, from hypnosis to biofeedback. There are two points that must be addressed in any of them. First, the underlying mechanism of relaxation is not necessarily reduced peripheral stress, reduced muscle firing, or reduced overall stress in biochemical reaction. More important, what effective relaxation therapies accomplish is a *transformation* of the pain image. They help the patient alter his or her perception of what pain is and is not. For example, patients who panic every time they see a syringe because they have learned to associate it with pain can, in a relaxed state, learn to reassociate the image with a new emotional response.

The second important aspect of relaxation is the generalization process. In order for the relaxation process to be beneficial, the patient needs to learn to desensitize to pain in situations beyond the relaxation therapy. If relaxation occurs only while listening to music or hearing soothing words from a therapist, the patient will become dependent on the quiet room and music. Thus it is necessary to help the patient learn to take the relaxation into other activities such as work, exercise, stretching, and walking, so that he or she can extend the altered pain image to other situations.

The transition from the solitude of the first relaxation phase to the activity desensitization phase is often accomplished in two steps. The image of relaxing while being active can be initiated through mental visualization in the safety of the relaxation room, which enables the patient to explore new realities in which to redefine pain. The second stage of the process involves introducing actual physical activity while maintaining the relaxation stimulus with headsets or portable biofeedback equipment. These help provide the cues necessary to help maintain the relaxation state when generalizing to other situations, especially when those situations have often been long associated with fear.

2. *Control techniques.* A very frequent feeling for many patients is helplessness and the loss of perceived control. Many hours of experience and research have supported the fact that positive changes in pain-management skills are effected through the teaching of perceived control.[13] Probably the most frequently used methods of gaining a sense of control over pain have been through controlled breathing techniques and biofeedback approaches. In regard to the latter, while it is true that if a person can raise his or her peripheral temperature, blood flow is increased and sympathetic stimulation is reduced, in fact it makes little difference whether the temperature goes up or down. What is significant is that the person feels that he or she has learned some control. It is the patient's sense of mastery over the situation that leads to the decrease in pain levels.

Being in a pediatric cancer clinic and teaching young children to deal with pain has reaffirmed my belief that the most effective way to teach mastery of pain is through breathing techniques. Children as young as two and three can learn the "blow" technique very easily, which renders them capable of dealing with very painful interventions with apparent ease. Altering a child's physiological perception also changes his or her entire experience of the world, thereby creating opportunities to reframe the whole process of healing in other realms. Of course, since children's boundaries between fantasy and reality are fluid and their images less rigidly formed than those of adults, they are easily taught pain-management techniques that are almost impossible for grownups. Nevertheless, breathing techniques are still the most powerful approaches for mastery of pain at any age.

3. *Finding meaning in pain.* Perhaps most relevant to adult patients of any cultural background is the issue of meaninglessness. As we have already seen, many of the associations to the experience of pain involve the emotional construct of shame and punishment. In addition, being in pain often entails the loss of role and social standing in the family and community. Introducing the concept that there may be meaning in the painful experience can be an antidote to these negative feelings. This can best be accomplished in group activities where there is a strong stense of community. In this context, we introduce the idea that the pain may present an opportunity for self-knowledge, insight, and personal growth. We have observed striking improvement if the patient can perceive meaning in his illness or injury. As Viktor Frankl observed with great clarity about his experiences in a concentration camp, the people who can invest meaningfulness in seemingly random horrible events can change their self-image from that of "victim" to that of someone who is "traveling a hero's journey."[14] As long as the person imagines him- or herself as a victim, he or she will stay a victim, to pain or to whatever else comes along.

Interview with Jeanne Achterberg, PH.D

Author of *Imagery in Healing* and *Woman as Healer*

Frank Lawlis: In your clinical work and research on pain, what relevance do you see for transpersonal medicine?

Jeanne Achterberg: First of all, there is an obvious medical application using an altered state of consciousness that is, unfortunately, almost never employed. In cases of severe or intractable pain, such as is experienced by severely burn-injured individuals, postoperative pain, and pain associated with some forms of cancer, major pain medications such as the opiates are normally administered—as they should be if needed. These very same medications—and other plant substances with narcotic properties—have historically and cross-culturally been highly prized and used as part of spiritual practices. They are believed to assist in communion with spirits and with the inner reaches of self. In ceremonial settings they are used by healers and those seeking healing and for traveling to other realms for power and information. Some can argue that such practices are inappropriate and dangerous for modern cultures, but that is not the point at all. They are already being used with great regularity in hospitals. I always suggest to my patients that they ask for and accept pain medication when needed, and then I give them the information I just gave you—giving them the opportunity to use the experience in a deeper sense. I also remind them to work (or "ride") with the effect of the drugs—often they fight them, fear them, feel like failures for needing them—and allow themselves to dissociate, to travel out of their bodies wherever they want to go.

As an aside, people who are undergoing general anesthesia for surgery can also use this information. The state of consciousness anesthesia engenders is very unusual, life is almost suspended, and I can't help but think that it might be a great opportunity to survey the territory so close to the edge of being.

FL: Do you think all efforts should be made to reduce severe pain, or do you believe, as we often hear, that pain is a teacher and has a message that needs to be heard? Some therapists suggest that pain should even be exacerbated until its message pops out loud and clear.

JA: I do hear that also, and mostly from people who have not witnessed significant physical suffering. I remember doing a study on the pediatric oncology unit once, trying to find nonpharmacological ways to manage the children's pain during treatment procedures. (Incidentally, the best strategy was a combination of Lamaze breathing and music of their choice.) Anyway, the doctor was one of the most supportive I have ever worked with. I asked him why he took such an interest in the study, and he said that in his thirty years of experience he had seen that children never, never die peacefully, or in any way that a caring soul would wish upon them, unless their pain is managed. Severe, unending pain, whether it be of a mental, physical, or spiritual nature, serves no good purpose in my mind, and to say otherwise, I think, borders on ignorance or sadism.

So, I need to anchor one end of your question with that comment. On the other hand, I suppose everything has a message, a potential lesson. Pain, not the kind we've just talked about, but pain in its many dimensions, accelerates transformation, self-knowing, decision-making, priority-setting, you name it. We seem to limp along our life course, taking things for granted, ignoring the subtle voice to grow up, transcend, move on—until we are stung by some kind of arrow that says, "Pay attention."

Would you allow anyone who had not experienced challenges (a nice word for pain) in some dimension to give you advice on how to live your own life? Would you trust even a religious teacher who had only encountered bliss?

FL: I am not sure I would. Do you think this is where the concept of the "wounded healer" comes from?

JA: Yes. The wounded healer is an idea supposedly derived from tribal cultures where the vocation of healing typically emerges out of pain, disease, or a serious and long dark night of the soul. In order to heal, particularly for disease of the spirit (such as soul loss), the healers would not be trusted unless they had, themselves, come close to death and were reborn with the knowledge of how to pull people back over the threshold into the land of the living.

FL: On a more practical level, what do you see as the relationship between mind/body techniques, such as imagery, and pain?

JA: Pain does have a vital, lifesaving, undeniable purpose, and that is to signal to consciousness where the problem is. When people are using imagery for physical healing, I believe they succeed best if they direct or hold mind-stuff or consciousness in the place in the body where the disease resides. Said another way, imagery doesn't work well if a little movie is played out behind the eyes, but rather when the stream of attention is actually moved and held in the place calling for help. Sometimes this attention is all that is necessary. Several pain researchers have noted that as many as one-third of chronic pain patients experience total and complete relief simply by paying full attention like this. Even for headache pain, if you can hold attention in the pain, it seems to go away for the time being.

ɪɪɪ 11 ɪɪɪ

A CASE STUDY
OF RITUAL
HEALING

THIS IS THE STORY of a patient named B.E., whose narrative reflects the courage and insights that can arise along the path toward health. Like all such stories, this one is incomplete because life always brings new challenges. But this story conveys some very important points that have already been presented in this book. B.E.'s is a voice that speaks to us about the power of a loving community, the power of symbols and imagery, and the successful adventure of an individual who had the spirit and strength to jump into the darkness of the night and reach for a transformation.

B.E.'s Story

Part One: My History of Cancer and Discovery

I began chemotherapy treatment for multiple myeloma in April of 1991. This rare form of blood cancer had first been diagnosed in me eleven years earlier. My internist found a worrisome blip in a routine blood test and referred me to an oncologist, who made the diagnosis by bone marrow aspiration. In this procedure, some bone marrow is drawn out through a hollow needle pounded into the hip area of the pelvis. At that time the myeloma proved to be at a very early stage and the doctor did not recommend treatment, but rather that we keep a watchful eye on it.

The diagnosis frightened me. My wife and grown children were frightened too, and we had a few sessions of family therapy together to help us talk about our feelings. My wife and I did a number of things to try to help me. I got her to help me change my diet in a Pritikin direction (this was before the American Cancer Society was ready to recognize any link between diet and cancer). We also planned some ways to reduce my work stress.

I read as much as I could find about this disease. Because it is a fairly rare form of cancer, the literature is not extensive. I learned that multiple myeloma affects the white blood cells in the bone marrow. Because white cells are major players in the immune system, the progression of the disease eventually compromises the immune system and leaves the body susceptible to other infections and diseases. As the cancer cells multiply in the bone marrow, they also crowd out the other healthy white cells and red cells and, in time, penetrate the interior of the bone itself with tumors that weaken the bones' structure. The disease is considered incurable, though not untreatable. Doctors don't know of any patient who has not in time died of this disease, but its course can be extremely variable. About half of patients respond well to treatment, which is usually oral chemotheraphy.

Multiple myeloma has the interesting property of sometimes lying "indolent" or "smoldering" for long periods of time. In my case the "indolent" period lasted eleven years. After the initial diagnosis, we followed the disease carefully with blood tests at frequent intervals. What shows up in the blood are not the cancer cells as such, but certain proteins called Bence Jones (after their discoverer) generated by those cells, which then provide something of an indicator of the activity of the cancer cells in the bone marrow. When those protein levels did not advance, but stayed steady month after month and then year after year, my anxiety about the myeloma subsided and I found it easier to accept my internist's hope that we were looking at a benign condition that sometimes imitates myeloma.

However, that more placid state of affairs came to an abrupt end in February of 1991 when a routine blood test for my annual physical exam showed a marked jump in the protein level. So I made another visit to the oncologist, had another bone marrow aspiration, and received confirmation that the myeloma now was becoming active.

Bemused by that medical term "indolent," I wrote to some friends about that time:

> It's as if I had this lazy, good-for-nothing son of a bitch lying around on the back porch, swigging corn whiskey and swatting flies—no good to anybody but not much harm either. Now after eleven years he has roused up, decided to get active, is stomping around in the garden messing things up, and scaring the hell out of me. I'm trying to figure out how to get him to lie down and be lazy again.

My own knowledge of that ominous secret brought heavy waves of sadness and fear for a time. The first day home from the oncologist's office, my wife and I sat on the couch and held each other and wept. A few days later I sat in my office leading a therapy group filled with people I had come to know and cherish over a long period of time. Grief filled my chest and squeezed my heart. It was as if I were already having to say goodbye to these people I loved.

About fear: I had the awesome experience of being held and supported as I plunged all the way, I think, to the bottom of my terror. It happened in Group 17. Group 17 is an extraordinary therapy group to which I have belonged as a patient for nearly twenty years.

This meeting was early in March of 1991, soon after the ominous signal in the blood profile, and before the bone marrow diagnosis. So I was in a confused and wobbly emotional state, which I tried to describe to the group. Sitting next to me was a dear friend who herself has had much acquaintance with physical illness and suffering. She kept gently and persistently pushing through my words, in search of what was behind them. I am unable to recall much content of that conversation, but I got closer and closer to my fear, which seemed to be about *helplessness*. I remember asking her, in a voice beginning to choke with tears, "What can I do?" Gravely she replied, "I don't know what to tell you to do, but I can tell you that I love you." My eyes closed and the tears poured. As best I can describe the experience of the next few moments, I think I went down into a place of absolute helplessness and vulnerability. I was exposed and utterly naked. I didn't have a thing to hold on to or cover myself with.

Amazingly, it was all right to be there. It was as if I had gone all the way to the bottom of whatever this terror was and found that I could survive. I didn't explode, or implode, or blow away, or melt, or burn up. I found I could just be there. It also becomes clearer, as I look back on this experience, that my deepest fear seems not to be about death, but about vulnerability and helplessness, nakedness.

I don't remember how long I stayed in that power circle, but I know it to be one of the deep healing experiences of my life. Later I said, "Boy, if that circle were a machine I could get hooked up to in the doctor's office, it would cost a thousand dollars a minute."

In addition to Group 17, I happened to have a good personal therapist at hand. J. is a gifted neurolinguistic programming teacher and therapist, and I have experience and credentials in marriage and family therapy. We each wanted to learn from the other, so we had set up a schedule to trade off teaching and consultation.

That process was just nicely under way when the roof fell in on me, and we changed the contract at my request. "I want your help in dealing with this crisis in my life," I said.

I was sitting in her office, puzzling aloud about the possible symbolic meaning of this strange cancer threatening my life. J. said, "Why don't you make an imaginary journey down inside your bone marrow and look around to see what you can find?" That is a process I am familiar with in my own personal pilgrimage and in my work with therapy clients, so I was readily able to imagine myself there in microscopic size inside my bone marrow. What I saw immediately were large, bulbous, soft, floating, papery, balloonlike figures, half-floating, half-bouncing along, coming at me in great numbers. Though slightly larger than I, they were light and easy to push aside or push back and, in fact, easy to puncture and deflate and had no apparent way of hurting me. Although I couldn't make out their danger to me, I began immediately to have the most uncanny, spooky, creepy, scared feeling. "I don't like it here," I thought, "I want to get out of here." Because I have learned from past experience that feelings like that are probably a clue to something important trying to get through to me, I also said, "I'd better stay here awhile and see what this is all about."

It didn't take long. It suddenly came to me that these white bulbous figures were female forms! It occurred to me later that they resembled the Venus of Willendorf, that famous prehistoric fertility symbol, headless and limbless, all breasts, belly, and buttocks. In my imagery, these figures were papery and soft, rather than made of stone, but they certainly were female forms.

"My God, J.," I said. "Here is the story of my life, coping with the powerful, overwhelming female. Why is that now being acted out in my bone marrow?"

You will not be surprised, if you know how these things work, to learn that I had fallen in love with and married a woman strong, warm, and passionate, who turned out to have a great capacity for anger. The anger didn't show at first, but I began very artfully to elicit it after a year or so into the marriage, by playing my father's game of being passive and avoidant. My wife, too, needed a partner to meet her at the emotional level, and when I, in my timidity, either avoided her or tried to placate her, her frustration and anger grew.

The results have been very interesting and gratifying. Though my wife sometimes winces at my fierceness, she likes my being present to her. It is as if her energy no longer sails out into a vacuum, but is being met by energy coming back from me. And at that meeting place a lot of life, love, and fun are generated. I have also learned that sometimes her anger is a mask for pain, and that if I simply put my arms around her and hold her lovingly, she "melts" and accepts comforting from me.

This has clearly been a major theme in our life together, and an important theme in my development as a person and a man. The successful work that we have done in realigning our relationship has had creative implications for my other relationships—to our children, to my clients, to students, colleagues, and friends. It has made a great difference to me, one that I am both grateful for and proud of.

So now I am back here in my bone marrow with this stunning discovery. I thought I had this issue resolved, and now at the very cellular level of my body, it seems to be coming at me again in an ominous and deadly way. These female figures, these bulbous cells, are out to do me in.

Group 17 urged me to develop a warrior image to do battle against these dangerous cancer cells. I came up with an image of myself as a kind of Robin Hood, with a special sword with a magic tip that could puncture and deflate a cell easily, as well as having a sharp edge that could cut through the papery form of the cells with no trouble. I bought a skeletal chart showing the areas of the bones where the myeloma would most likely be active and set about a kind of systematic sweep. In my mind's eye, I would cut and slash my way through hundreds or thousands of these white cells, leaving their tattered remnants on the ground. But it wasn't long before I began to have trouble with this imagery work, and the trouble was that I got tired. Even though this work was all in my imagination, the very notion of swinging that sword around and back and forth for hours on end brought on an imagined but real fatigue. And in addition to that, these cells had a discouraging propensity for reassembling and re-forming behind me not long after I had swept an area clean. It was like trying to sweep out the ocean. I was back, talking about my discouragement about staying at this kind of imagery work, when it suddenly dawned on me, and I said aloud, "I am not using my best resource for this work. I'm not using my 'Brute.' "

Here I need to make another detour to introduce "Brute." Some years ago in a guided imagery workshop, I encountered what I could call a lost part of myself. I came upon a strange figure nailed shut in a rough-hewn box, about four feet on each side. As I peered into the darkness of the box, it seemed to contain a kind of primitive, hairy, apelike creature. Later I thought of his similarity to Robert Bly's "Iron John," the hairy man at the bottom of the pond. Here is some kind of archetypal figure of primitive masculine power that my father did not know how to access in himself and therefore did not know how to introduce me to. So I had him, as it were, nailed shut in this big old box, and it was exciting and scary to discover him. But one of the most exciting experiences in all my years with that group was the day I took my primitive friend around the circle and introduced him to each of the members. That is also where his name came from, because when I asked his name, the word "Brute" came to my tongue unbidden.

Back to my imagery work: I realized that I was failing to use a part of myself that ought to be helpful. So I summoned Brute, and the result of that was fascinating. It turns out that Brute takes to this job with zest and gusto. What he does is to grab three or four or five of these big inflated figures in a great bear hug and squeeze them, and all the air goes out of them in a big "whoosh," and they collapse and slide to the ground. Then he grabs some more and repeats the process. He loves doing that, and he does it without fatigue and, apparently, without rest. Whenever I check in with him, he is busy hugging and squeezing and deflating bunches of cells and is more than able to stay ahead of them, no matter how fast they are reproducing. When I want a workout, I can go down there and join him and grab one or two of these cells myself and give them a big squeeze, and listen as the air goes out with a big *whoosh*, and the remnants slide to the ground. Brute and I then grin at each other and have at it for a while, and then I bid him good hunting and take off to attend to other matters.

I came across an audiotape of a workshop that had been presented by Jeanne Achterberg and Frank Lawlis in which they were talking about imagery and healing. This is an area in which the two of them have done a lot of interesting work. I had met each of them briefly in the past and had read their books and was now reminded that they might be excellent resources for me in trying to clarify and develop what felt like unfinished parts of my imagery work here. I enrolled in a weekend workshop on imagery and healing in late May.

About twenty people were in our group that weekend, and Frank and Jeanne introduced us to a number of interesting modes of facilitating healing—through use of sound and movement and group ritual and other aspects of what they generally described as "shamanic resources."

At one point, Frank came and stood beside me and guided me into a couple of new experiences, the second of which turned out to be astonishing. First, he had me close my eyes and rock back and forth from one foot to the other; he stood beside me and rocked with me with one arm around me. The rocking had a kind of rhythmic quality, and he invited me to go into my healing scene and watch what happened. It fit very nicely with the scene in which Brute is carrying out his campaign, because the rocking felt a little like marching in place as in a military operation; Brute and I found that rhythm worked very well in our crushing the white cancer cells.

Then I flashed upon another scene that I had once imagined, what I call the "nativity scene." Here the rocking seemed very much out of place. The mother and infant in this scene are very quiet, in gentle repose, and for me to be standing there rocking back and forth felt like a kind of agitation, a nervous twitch. So that didn't fit. I opened my eyes and reported this to Frank and the group.

This time he had me place one hand on my stomach and the other on my upper chest, and he placed a hand on each of mine. He asked me to close my eyes and begin to hum. I started off humming at a fairly deep note. ("Let's make this a 'manly' hum.") Each time I would take a breath and start a new hum, I raised the pitch a bit. I discovered that I could keep the tone going longer with a higher pitch, so over several breaths I raised the pitch, step by step. I could feel my energy rising as I was doing this, and later Frank reported that, as he was humming along with me, he could at the beginning hold a breath through two of mine, but, by the time I finished, he was breathing twice for each one of my breaths.

What I saw happening in my mind's eye as I was humming seemed to me quite wonderful. I was standing by the mother and baby and singing to this newborn child. I was singing to him about what it means to be a man in this world. I don't know any of the verbal content, but I was singing to him very precious information, all the things that he would need to know to make his way in the world. This infant child could be my son, or it could be my own infant self; but I was singing him into his being.

I am reminded, as I think about this, of Bruce Chatwin's writings about the Australian aborigines who sing enormously elaborate songs that are in effect maps of vast stretches of their territory, and who say that their forefathers "sang the world into being."

So I am singing this newborn into his being. I said later to Frank that my father didn't sing to me; I'm not sure that I sang very well to my own sons and daughter. I'm not sure altogether yet what that means—to sing or not sing to one's children. But it feels like a powerful metaphor for something that a father needs to transmit to his children.

As I am singing, I notice something else happening. The energy of my song is flowing into these other cells that have been lying inert against that back wall. They begin to glow, and they begin to buzz, and they begin to move—to lift, to bounce and jump and fly about. Hosts of them begin to fly this way and that. Some of them go to where the empty husks of the old cancer cells are lying on the ground and, like Pac-men, gobble them up. I had wondered previously how those empty husks were going to be disposed of, and now I found out. I could feel, as it were, this sort of buzzing energy flowing through my whole body, coming alive, vibrating with a wonderful zip.

So I came back from that experience feeling energized and alive in a new way, and I can recover that sense of live energy pulsing through my body whenever I bring that scene to mind, whenever I revisualize that experience.

I then decided that I would go back for the five-day workshop offered by Jeanne and Frank at Esalen in August. This time I had a less clear agenda, since I felt that I had accomplished my goal the first time in finding a way to round out my incomplete imagery work. But I was intrigued by other things that Frank and Jeanne were offering in their shamanic rituals, and I thought it a good investment to have another round with them. What happened this time was less dramatic, in terms of new insight, but very powerful in terms of a new kind of communal experience for me.

About twenty people were also in this workshop, only one of whom had been in the other, so Frank invited me to tell the group about my cancer and about my imagery work. They seemed fascinated by my account and were quite ready to participate in a healing ritual that Frank and Jeanne set up for us:

I was asked to stand in the middle of the room with Frank close by my side, and the members of the group gathered around. They were invited to touch or pat me in whatever ways seemed loving and appropriate for them and to join me as I closed my eyes and started humming again. The humming filled the room with marvelous sound. We played with varying pitches and harmonies, and the volume and energy grew and grew. Then I found I could no longer contain the sound within me behind closed lips, so I opened my mouth and let the sound come out and soar up toward the ceiling. I am still not sure how to describe the sound I heard, or if there is any one word to characterize it. It was high-pitched, with some of the quality of a scream, something like a wail, something like a yell of triumph, something like a battle cry. Other mouths opened and voices joined mine and rocked the room. I thought afterwards that that first cry from me might have been like the anguished cry of a newborn infant, outraged at being thrust into the world where he has to breathe and fend for himself. But it flowed quickly into becoming some kind of triumphant sound, a victory cry, a warrior's exultation. As the group milled around me, joining in the cry, patting and touching me, sharing in a triumphal song, I began to feel like a newborn being welcomed into a sacred tribe. All these people were my parents, my siblings, my grandparents, my cousins, my nephews and nieces, my distant relatives, all united in kinship and love, giving thanks for my birth, welcoming me and singing me into my new life, celebrating the miracle of birth and life.

So I returned from my workshop with a richer and deeper gift. When I take myself in memory back into that experience, I can both feel and hear within my body and spirit this pulsing song of life. It is a song I am singing, and it is a song being sung to me and through me by my sacred tribal family.

I think it is an interesting story, one that is important for my life. Is it—or could it be—important for anyone else? That is the question I put to my Esalen family group. They replied with a kind of urgent consensus: "Don't you realize how valuable it has been for us to hear this story just as you have told it?" I answered: "If you tell me that, I believe it; but I am still not clear how that happens, how it is useful to you."

Nevertheless, I have undertaken to put it here on paper, and to send it forth on whatever voyage it may take. In Part Two of this account to follow, I will offer some thoughts of my own about this narrative.

Part Two: My Reflections on the Process

Some obvious questions are: Does this imagery ritual work have any discernible effect on the medical course of my cancer? Is it helping me get well or stay well?

An honest answer has to be that I believe so but do not know. As of this writing (October 1992) my protein level is coming down significantly, indicating that the cancer is for now in retreat. Unhappily, my healthy white cell count also tends to dip down to the danger level, where the doctor worries about my immune system. So for now we are easing back on the amount of chemotherapy. In terms of my imagery work, it is as if Brute were doing his job well, but I need to put more attention and energy into "singing" my healthy cells alive and active. So I have become more disciplined about that recently.

I was also reminded that I have not yet described in my narrative how I visualized the chemotherapy working in my body. Then I realized that all this vivid imagery of healing did not somehow include the chemotherapy process. How does it fit in there?

The answer did not come quickly. But after waiting patiently for a minute or two, I began to see a kind of silver rain drifting down from above. On closer examination I could see little icy discs with jagged edges, spinning down. As they struck the papery cancer cells, they cut through them easily and left them deflated and limp.

In the other, what I have called the nativity scene, the damage from these discs was mitigated by two factors. First, the warm golden light bathing this scene melts the jagged edges of the icy discs so they don't cut as sharply. Secondly, the vulnerable infant's body is sheltered by the mother's body and, to some extent, the father's, who suffers some bruises and welts but not lethal cuts.

Back to the question of how this mental work affects what goes on in my body. We may never know the answer to that in any convincing way. My oncologist is pleased about the retreat of the cancer and sees it as a not unusual result of the course of chemotherapy. He is benignly skeptical about psychosocial interventions of the kind I have described here and cautions me not to build my hopes on such practices.

The potential of the relation of body and spirit is so rich and complex as to defy simple formulae. But I can identify two positions I believe to be clearly wrong. The first is based on the classic Cartesian split between body and the spirit/mind. In this view, which essentially underlies Western scientific medicine, the body is a complicated machine running by its own rules. It is affected by intruders like germs and viruses, and by internal malfunctions, but not by attitudes, emotions, or intentions of the person-in-the-body.

That view is getting tougher for all but the most zealous medical technician to hold. Floods of information about such matters as placebo effect, plus newer research on psychoneuroimmunology, added to anecdotal accounts from all ages of medicine, tell us that the Cartesian boundary is indeed very porous. It leaks copiously in both directions.

But there is an equally preposterous position that oversimplifies that complex body-mind relationship in the opposite direction, holding that the body is a kind of extension of the mind without its own autonomy. Christian Science is a traditional example of this view, but it has been showing up in a number of New Age cosmologies. One wills one's illness (though perhaps unconsciously) and thus can will it away. If I change my attitude, image the right images, pray the right prayers, meditate the right meditations, I can make the deadliest disease go away.

If I don't succeed in that, it means that I didn't do it right. So I get to bear the double onus of having made myself ill and then failing to make myself well.

Both of these extreme positions seem to me preposterous or bizarre. Somewhere in between is the great fascinating area of mystery and possibility.

Is my imagery work effective in healing my cancer? I believe so, but at this point I don't know how to demonstrate that. What I do know is that it is *healing for me as a person*, in very important ways.

First of all, it gives me something to *do*, to be an active participant in my own healing process. To feel helpless, totally dependent on the power of another to preserve or protect one's life, is scary and demoralizing. There may be some for whom that is a comforting place, who feel so burdened and defeated by life that it is a relief to turn the whole responsibility for it over to another, but I do not count myself among them.

When I had heart bypass surgery three years ago, I was by necessity in that kind of helpless place for a while, and I believe I managed it with some grace. In the recovery room I could do little for myself. I even had a machine with a tube down my throat to breathe for me. It wasn't easy, but I accepted my essential helplessness and dependency on the competence and goodwill of the people assigned to care for me.

While life on occasion may deal us a hand like that, I don't have to see my cancer that way—a game in which the doctor has some cards to play, but I have none. I am going to play the cards I can find. What kind of game is this? This question brings me to the second aspect of my imagery work—the more interesting and puzzling issue.

If this is a *lesson* I haven't finished learning, who or what sends the lesson? None of the available answers to that question make much sense to me. I don't see God sending the cancer for punitive or pedagogical reasons. Nor does it make sense to me to say that I brought this cancer on myself. All I know is that I am presented in a new way with a picture of a major drama in my life, and I have the opportunity to engage with it with as much vigor, courage, and imagination as I can muster.

A larger question could be asked at this point. Even if we grant, as I am disposed to do, that there is a significant relation between the form of my cancer and the "form" of my life, is there anything generalizable about that, anything applicable to someone else's cancer or someone else's life?

I would like to believe so, but I still have many more questions than answers about it. For example, do other multiple myeloma patients have life issues like mine with the powerful female? I would be fascinated, but also I think surprised, to learn that that was true.

There is a double area of mystery here, with far more questions than answers. There is the area of *meaning*. My cancer seems a metaphor for important dimensions of my life: Is that true for others? And there is the dimension of *healing*. What heals? And how?

I don't know the answers to those questions, but I ponder some of the ironies around the healing issue. The language of cancer treatment is replete with military metaphors—the "war" or "battle" against cancer. We have been in an official government-sponsored "War Against Cancer" for some twenty years. (Except for some notable small victories, the overall story is that we are losing.)

But if the struggle with cancer is a war, it is a strange war. One of the things we know about cancer is that it is an aspect of the *life process gone awry*. Cancer cells proliferate and multiply out of control. Normal cells respond to chemical signals telling them when to slow down or stop reproduction. In cancer cells the stop or slow-down signals don't work, and the unlimited growth fills up (in my case, literally) space needed for other healthy processes and thereby becomes destructive.

So from the very beginning of my visualization work, I pondered the ambiguity of calling this cancer an enemy. In an obvious sense, it is an enemy, a killer, that in the expected course of the disease will wind up killing me sooner or later. So I ought to do what I can to kill it instead.

That, by the way, is what the chemotherapy is about: it is a poison that attacks all the cells in the body. Cells are most vulnerable when they are dividing, and cancer cells divide more quickly than healthy cells. Thus the right dosage of poison knocks off lots of cancer cells with tolerable damage to healthy cells. In those terms it certainly sounds like a war: kill them before they kill you.

But the battlefield imagery has never quite felt right to me. Cancer may kill, but calling it a killer is something different. "Life force gone out of control" sounds truer.

Brute's tireless assault on the cancer cells looks somewhat like a battlefield, strewn with corpses. But the battle is an odd one, as much playful as warlike. When the air goes out of those balloon figures and they collapse, they certainly change in a dramatic way, but I am not sure the change is from life to death.

I am remembering now that I did find myself in a more bloody kind of battle imagery with my cancer. While I was told that my imagery and resources were very impressive, perhaps I was too gentle. Did I have the guts to do real battle with this cancer? "It's not being gentle with you," J. said. "It seems as if it is out to kill you."

That caught my attention, and I settled into another internal imagery journey. What emerged was a scene dimly lit by a red "bloody" light, in the back of the stage of my mind's eye, behind and between the other two scenes. Seated there was Medusa, with snaky hair and a face to turn a man to stone. Perseus had been crafty enough to use his polished shield as a mirror, in order to get close enough to Medusa to behead her.

In my scene I was luckier, if not craftier, than Perseus, because, as Medusa was looking to the right, I was able to sneak up behind her on the left, swing my great sword, and chop off her head before she could turn. It was a great moment of triumph, but it was followed by an even greater one.

In my left hand I picked up Medusa's head—her dead face no longer toxic—by the still-squirming snakes, and holding my bloody sword aloft in the right, I advanced to the front of the stage. It turned out to be indeed a theater, with footlights and a great audience of hundreds facing me and rising now to give me a standing ovation. What a moment of exaltation!

That scene is exciting to remember and write about, but I am still not sure what to make of it. It does not feel as organically a part of me as do the other two scenes. I might lack the spleen to kill if my life depended on it. From another perspective I can see and grin at my narcissistic exhibitionism here—anything for a standing ovation!

As for killing the cancer, I am still uncomfortable with that language. The cancer cells are a part of me that once worked to protect my life. They have lost direction and control and are now banging around inside in a way dangerous and ultimately lethal to me.

Perhaps there is a piece of imagery yet to emerge. Maybe it will show the cancer cells recycling into healthy forms. If that happens, it will certainly be consistent with my experience as a psychotherapist dealing with unwanted interjects, in myself or others. Clients often come to the therapist with the request to help them get rid of something they despise or abhor in themselves—and I have been that route myself. What I have learned is that therapy usually doesn't work that way. It is rather the other way around. What I try to get rid of tends to cling like Velcro—and what I try to hold on to slips away between my fingers. True therapy is about opening up and adding things, not about contracting and amputating things. It usually proceeds by having the courage to own and embrace the rejected part, the *shadow* in Jungian terms.

It sounds as if I were trying to find a way to "embrace" my cancer. That may be true. In my personal reflection, and in my reading of other persons' accounts of their struggles with mortal illness, I have more and more come to find a profound polarity here—a polarity, a dialectic, or a paradox—something with two opposite faces, both true. The polarity is between "fighting against" on the one hand, and "accepting" or "flowing with" on the other. Between "pushing away" and "embracing." Between turning away from and turning toward. These pairs seem contradictory, in a logical sense, but somehow true to the dialectical dance of the healing process, as I experience it.

I remember one night early in my treatment when I was in a somewhat anguished quest for a way to orient myself to this illness, and I awoke in the middle of the night. A sentence had come into my consciousness: "I am not willing to make death an enemy, nor dying a defeat." I don't know where those words came from, but they soothed my troubled spirit, and I relaxed and went back to sleep.

Eastern religions like Buddhism see *attachment* as the major source of human suffering. We can be attached to something either positively or negatively. If positively, we try to hold on to it, defining our happiness or well-being in terms of its possession; if negatively, we try to avoid or get rid of it, thus defining our well-being in terms of our *not* having it (as, for example, an illness).

In bringing this essay to a close, at least for now, I want to try to make more explicit some ideas I see bubbling to the surface in what I have been writing.

1. Healing is not defined by "cure." Healing means "making whole," and it can embrace one's dying.
2. The only space and time for living is in the here and now. Each moment can be welcomed as a miracle.

3. True wisdom is to know that "everything is interesting and nothing is important."

At present, my cancer appears to be in retreat, with my doctor and I winning the current battle, if not the war. I am pleased about that, and hopeful about living several more productive years. But I have no way of knowing how many years there will be, and I am not terribly concerned about that. This confrontation with my mortality has reawakened for me the knowledge that I can live only in the present, and that each day is itself a gift and a miracle. I like what Anatole Broyard said of facing his dying (from prostate cancer): "The wonder and the terror and the exaltation of being at the edge of being."

COMMENTARY

I included B.E.'s story as a tribute to his courage and insight into the healing process. In his words the elements of transpersonal medicine reveal themselves in a natural flow, manifesting the potential relationships of the body-mind-spirit through the imagerial material. The healing process happens through the pilgrimage of learning and exploring the totality of life, including the family, community, and personal history. Within a multi-layered reality, B.E. has described his healing story in his own terms.

In B.E.'s story arise many questions common to those who have been diagnosed with a life-threatening condition: Is this disease my special path? Is the form of my disease a reflection of the form of my life? Will I get well if I do this or that? The answers to these questions—persistent since the beginning of time—are beyond rational intelligence.

However, as B.E. continues to describe his search and articulate his progress to us, we begin to catch a glimpse of the mystery hidden in each of us and of the empowerment we can receive from those around us. We watch as B.E. opens doors into altered states of consciousness, behind which he finds new avenues to symbols in healing. We see him use the imagery process with its exquisite power and intention as well as its vivid insight into the dynamics of the many aspects of disease and health. We meet his co-consciousness, personified by Brute and the figure of Medusa, coming forth, ready to inject new power and strength into B.E.'s healing.

In addition, B.E.'s descriptions of his encounters with Group 17 and his Esalen family convey the potentials of transpersonal imagery, relationship, and rituals to empower and enhance healing. After writing a book about transpersonal medicine in which its components by necessity had to be broken into topics and addressed with linear thinking, I am grateful to B.E. for presenting such a rich, succinct, and clear expression of the underlying root of this approach—the "oneness" of the human spirit.

One of the major features of his story is the description of his attitude in the last paragraph. He says, "I have no way of knowing how many years there will be, and I am not terribly concerned about that." In all the patients with whom I have worked, the most important determinant of how well they will do physically, psychologically, and spiritually is framed in those words related to their potential life span: "I am not terribly concerned about that." The onset of disease is usually a threatening call to arms, with the dire prognosis articulated in terms of time units (six months, two years, and so on). When the patient releases that concept of time and space into one of true connectedness with the universe and embraces the day-to-day experience of being in the present, I know that true healing has occurred. When a patient can say that the unfolding of the present moment is the most important part of their lives, that they feel joy in the here and now, that all regrets or guilts are released, then I know that the cure has happened. This state of being is well expressed in the Native American affirmation, "Today is a good day to die."

This statement articulates the state in which all is complete and beautiful, there are no attachments, and the return to the cosmos in true energy form can be celebrated without hope or fear. Would that all of my transitions could be that smooth, that I would have no fear or hesitation to enter whatever sphere of consciousness the universe requires of me, but I am not yet that evolved. However, I have learned from my teachers, particularly my patients, that true happiness is the wholeness that allows for such transformation. If I can trust each day and the wisdom of the universe, I will be blessed.

EPILOGUE

The week that I completed the last major revision of this book, I experienced a major event that offered me the ultimate opportunity to become a true healer, to myself.

After teaching a morning class on imagery, I began to have very strange sensations throughout my body. My vision was impaired, as if I were in a dark tunnel. At that moment I experienced a heart attack and lost consciousness.

I awoke to the sight of medics attaching an I.V. bottle to my arm. They took me to the emergency room at Stanford Hospital, where they checked out my EKG readings and blood levels. After some deliberation and a thousand questions, I was sent to the Cardiac Intensive Care Unit, although at that time no one was sure what had happened to me. My EKG was normal, my blood levels were good. The only concern was a very low pulse rate and low blood pressure.

The angiography studies conducted the next day revealed a blockage of the right coronary artery and a partial blockage of the anterior descending branch of the left coronary artery. The blockage in the right artery, probably due to a blood clot, explained the sudden loss of blood pressure and restricted flow to the brain, which resulted in loss of consciousness. I agreed to an immediate angioplasty procedure in which the team broke through the blockage and expanded that region.

The results of the procedure were gratifying. My blood pressure and pulse rate returned to normal. I passed a stress test on the treadmill and an echocardiogram and was released four days after the event. However, there was grave concern over my projected rehabilitation. The anterior descending artery is more critical to survival, and the medical team expressed their strong recommendation that we conduct another angioplasty procedure quickly to open up this passage, which was 80 percent blocked. However, there are dangers associated with this process, and knowing that it might take six months for the artery to completely block up, I wanted to try my healing path first.

Dr. John Schroeder and I agreed that I would return for a thallium stress test in two weeks and assess the ongoing problems. I would make a decision at that time as to the potential risk and whether or not my program was working.

My Program

To summarize the journey I set out for myself would be to review every chapter of this book. I focused upon meditation, imagery, exercise, lifestyle, ritual, humor, and community support. Although none of these components were independent from the others, the one I felt most strongly was community support.

I have never felt so much love and care in my life. Healing circles were set up for me virtually all over the world. I received hundreds of calls, cards, and gifts, and each one touched me in a specific and wonderful way. My son came to help me, and my sister flew in with her care and concern.

Relationships were healed and celebrated. My spirit soared with each interaction and touch. The love shared with each individual was more than a sense of entitlement or mere exchange of caring responses. I began to experience it as a pure blessing and grace with no attempt to justify what was happening to me nor to understand it. This was my healing path.

My imagery was of honeybees collecting the plaque from my blood vessels, opening them to greater flow. The important dimension I discovered was their motivation. They were motivated by love for me, increased by the network of those marvelous friends and family members who cared.

The lifestyle changes were my greatest challenge. But fortunately, Jeanne's talents are not restricted to academics. She moved to the kitchen and masterfully shifted my diet to nonfat (less than 10 percent). My cholesterol levels have always been less than 150, so I did not fit the profile for a heart attack; nevertheless, I was overweight, and I felt that I needed to communicate with my body on all levels. Therefore, Dean Ornish's books became our consultation and guides.

But work is my passion, so I needed help in this area badly. In several vision quests, the spirit guides were very clear—too many time zone changes, too fast. I also have a tendency to plan my life quickly and move directly forward. The message was: go with the flow, no plans, be present day by day. So I began to walk more on the earth with softer feet, more present intentions, allowing the river of life to flow without help.

In my life some of the most satisfying of my relationships have been within the business realm. My relationship with Jeanne began in business, most of my best friendships grew from business, and my fondest memories are within those communities that were formed with a missionary concept. I even developed business relationships with my children in order to experience that aspect of identification and companionship with them.

However, now I became aware of the fear associated with my business life. While my son was driving me home from the hospital, we were discussing the interesting relationships we had with our respective fathers. I realized that, through an early perception of my father, I have carried a deep fear of business failure, and that I use my many business interests to afford me some false sense of security. As I was expressing some of these early experiences, my son turned to me with a puzzled look and said, "Dad, you *are* a success now, regardless of what happens. You cannot fail now."

A chill ran down my back and tears came to my eyes as I realized that he was right. In fact, he would be right for all of us from our first day of life. We are successful; fear is not a healthy source of motivation.

But insight is not enough sometimes; it takes action to make it real. So every day I try to be present with not acting out of fear, but to be clear as to the true meaningfulness any activity has for me.

THE SHAMAN VISITS

Not surprising to me was the fact that my shaman friends knew of my "event" on other levels, probably before I did. Michael Harner told me to expect him in a dream, and he came the next night. In the context of death and rebirth, I went through an initiation rite in which I felt challenged to bring health to myself. The dream affirmed my sense of crisis and the importance of finding the right path.

Other friends had dreams of my healing. Others focused upon sending a stream of love my way. Still others sent wonderful jokes and cartoons for me to laugh my way back to health. Friends visited in my dreams; rituals were held for me. My kids in the Kids for Kids program drew pictures of health images and sent them to me. I have all the cards and letters in my special basket and ritually reread them all and bask again in their nurturance. Every spiritual tradition has been expressed in these messages: Christian, Buddhist, Shinto, Hindu, Jewish, Sikh, and so on.

PROGRESS NOTE

Two weeks after my heart attack, I returned to Stanford for the thallium stress test. The results were encouraging: the anterior wall showed no abnormalities, and the stress test showed no abnormalities. This meant to me that the blood flow as getting through and that I was doing something right. In fact, Dr. Shroeder said for me to keep doing whatever I was doing, but he would want to see me again in three months. "After all, you do need to be watched," he cautioned.

What a celebration! What a time to consider the message and lessons! I embraced Western medicine, for certainly the acute care was important and began in the depths of that science. My friends and family were terrific, and I attribute my personal and long-term rehabilitation in large measure to the healing force of their "Era III" nonlocal influence.

It would be very easy to let the event go at this point. I have little or no heart muscle damage, and there are few other discernible effects of the heart attack, yet this has been a lesson, a powerful message for change. I will continue to listen for its direction. The rapid health response was due to the total intensity of the support and care I received, and in order for my improvement to be sustained I must take responsibility to continue the initiated life changes.

REFLECTION

I am grateful for this experience, and I can better understand why other cultures so respect a survivor. Through trauma and disease we learn so much about ourselves, tapping a vital source of courage in order to cope. This disease has touched me at multiple levels, and I imagine that more lessons await me. But, as my son explained, I am a success, regardless of what happens. There is no failure and, by now, no longer any fear of it harbored within me.

I have learned a great deal about the deeper application of transpersonal medicine to my own situation, and I have rediscovered the power of love in healing, not only for myself, but for the planet. I am convinced that this is the major constructive force in our world and that it works, not only through individuals, but through many communities and collectives. As it is gentle by nature, this force is usually more latent than hostile ones, but by its focused consensual goodness, it is our hope and redemption. For lack of any better name, the principle underlying this effect of love could be called "transpersonal medicine."

> > >

NOTES

Preface

1. Leonard Sagan, *The Health of Nations: True Cause of Sickness and Well-Being* (New York: Basic Books, 1989).

Chapter 1: Transpersonal Medicine

1. Jeanne Achterberg, "Transpersonal Medicine: A Proposed System of Healing," *ReVision* 14 (1992): 127.
2. Jeanne Achterberg, "Ritual: The Foundation for Transpersonal Medicine," *ReVision*, Vol. 14, no. 3 (1992): 158–64.
3. Larry Dossey, "What Does Illness mean?" *Alternative Therapies* 1, no. 3 (1995): 6–10.
4. Franz J. Ingelfinger, "Health: A Matter of Statistics of Feelings," *New England Journal of Medicine* 296 (1977): 448–49.

Chapter 2: Rituals

1. Jeanne Achterberg,"Ritual: The Foundation for Transpersonal Medicine," *ReVision* 14, no. 3 (1992): 158–64.
2. J. S. House, K. R. Landis, and D. Umberson, "Social Relationships and Health," *Science* (29 July 1988): 540–50.

3. Frank Lawlis, *The Four Relationship Factor Questionnaire* (Wichita, Kans.: Test Systems, 1974).

4. R. J. Gatchel and A. Baum, *An Introduction to Health Psychology* (Reading, Mass.: Addison-Wesley, 1983).

5. Ernest Rossi, *The Psychobiology of Mind-Body Healing* (New York: W. W. Norton & Co., 1986).

6. Barbara Peavey, G. Frank Lawlis, and A. Govern, "Biofeedback-Assisted Relaxation: Effect of Phagocytic Capacity," *Biofeedback and Self-Regulation* 10 (1985): 33–47.

7. Peter Salmon, "Psychological Factors in Surgical Stress: Implications for Management," *Clinical Psychology Review* 12, no. 7 (1992): 45–54.

8. G. Frank Lawlis, David Selby, Glen Hinnant, and Edward McCoy, "Reduction of Postoperative Pain Parameters by Presurgical Relaxation Instructions for Spinal Pain Patients," *Spine* 10 (1985): 163–71.

9. Lawrence LeShan, *The Medium, the Mystic, and the Physicist* (New York: Viking Press, 1974).

10. Jeanne Achterberg, "Ritual: The Foundation for Transpersonal Medicine," *ReVision* 14, no. 3 (1992): 158–64.

11. William Bridges, *Transitions: Making Sense of Life's Changes* (Boston: Addison-Wesley, 1980).

12. Joseph Campbell, *Creative Mythology* (New York: Penguin Group, 1976), p. 4.

Chapter 3: Transpersonal Imagery and Healing

1. C. Backster, "Evidence of a Primary Perception in Plant Life," *International Journal of Parapsychology* 10 (1968): 329.

2. Larry Dossey, *Recovering the Soul* (New York: Bantam Books, 1989).

3. K. Lin, L. Demonteverde, and I. Nuccio, "Religion, Healing and Mental Health among Filipino Americans," *International Journal of Mental Health* 19, no. 3 (1990): 40–44.

4. Merriam-Webster, *Ninth New Collegiate Dictionary* (Springfield, Mass.: Merriam-Webster, 1987).

5. A. Gragory, "Conformance Behaviour Involving Animal and Human Subjects," *European Journal of Parapsychology* 3 (1976): 36–50.

6. L. L. Vasiliev, *Experiments in Distant Influence* (New York: Dutton, 1976).

7. William Braud and Marilyn Schlitz, "Psychokinetic Influence on Electrodermal Activity," *Journal of Parapsychology* 47 (1983): 95–119.

8. M. C. Dillbeck, G. Landrith, and D. W. Orme-Johnson, "The Transcendental Meditation Program and Crime Rate Change in a Sample of Forty-eight Cities," *Journal of Crime and Justice* 4 (1981): 25–45.

9. *The Maharishi Effect* (Fairfield, Iowa: Maharishi International University Press, 1990).

10. William Braud, "Distant Mental Influence on Rate of Hemolysis of Human Red Blood Cells," *The Journal of the American Society for Psychical Research* 84, no. 1 (1990): 1–24.

11. P. J. Collipp, "The Efficacy of Prayer: A Triple-blind study," *Medical Times* 97, no. 5 (1969): 201–04.

12. R. C. Byrd, "Positive Therapeutic Effects of Intercessory Prayer in a Coronary Care Unit Population," *Southern Medical Journal* 81 (1988): 826–29.

13. M. Murphy and R. White, *The Psychic Side of Sports* (New York: Addison-Wesley, 1978).

Chapter 4: Resonance

1. Abraham Maslow, *Toward a Psychology of Being* (Princeton, N.J.: Van Nostrand, 1968).

2. Martin Buber, *I and Thou* (New York: Scribner, 1958), p. 6.

3. Richard Moss, *The I That Is We* (Berkeley: Celestial Arts, 1981), p. 36.

4. V. A. Larson, "An Exploration of Psychotherapeutic Resonance," *Psychotherapy*, Vol. 24, no. 3 (1987): 321–24.

5. Ibid., p. 323.

6. J. Grinberg-Zylberbaum, "The Syntergic Theory," *Frontier Perspectives* 4, no. 1 (1994): 25–30.

7. See R. Penrose, *Shadows of the Mind* (New York: Oxford University Press, 1994).

8. Mark Rider, "Mental Shifts and Resonance: Necessities for Healing?" *ReVision* 14, no. 3 (1992): 149–57.

9. Dean Ornish, *Dr. Dean Ornish's Program for Reversing Heart Disease* (New York: Random House, 1990).

10. Personal communication, San Francisco, August 1994.

Chapter 5: Altered States of Consciousness

1. A. Ludwig, "Altered States of Consciousness," *Altered States of Consciousness*, C. Tart, ed. (New York: Wiley, 1969).

2. D. Shapiro, "A Biofeedback Strategy in the Study of Consciousness," in N. E. Zinberg (ed.), *Alternate States of Consciousness* (New York: Macmillan, 1977), pp. 145–57.

3. C. Marsh, "A Framework for Describing Subjective States of Consciousness," in N. E. Zinberg (ed.), *Alternate States of Consciousness* (New York: Macmillan, 1977), pp. 121–44.

4. Charles Tart, "Putting the Pieces Together: A Conceptual Framework for Understanding Discrete States of Consciousness," in N. E. Zinberg (ed.), *Alternate States of Consciousness* (New York: Macmillan, 1977), pp. 158–219.

5. T. Oxman, P. Schnurr, G. Tucker, and G. Gala, "The Language of Altered States," *The Journal of Nervous and Mental Disease* 176, no. 7 (1988): 401–08.

6. J. Ehrenwald, "Psi Phenomena, Hemispheric Dominance and the Existential Shift," in B. Shepin and L. Coly (eds.), *Psi and States of Consciousness* (New York: Parapsychology Foundation, 1978), pp. 21–22.

7. C. Cade and F. Coxhead, *The Awakened Mind, Biofeedback, and the Development of Higher States of Awareness* (New York: Delacorte, 1979).

8. Melinda Maxfield, "The Journey of the Drum," *ReVision* 16, no. 4 (1994): 157–63.

9. C. Burney, *Solitary Confinement* (New York: Coward-McCann, 1952). E. Anderson, "Abnormal Mental States in Survivors," *Journal of the Royal Navy Medical Services* 28 (1942): 361–77.

10. R. Byrd, *Alone* (New York: G. P. Putnam Sons, 1938).

11. W. Heron, "The Pathology of Boredom," *Scientific American* 196 (1957): 52–56.

12. P. Leiderman, "Imagery and Sensory Deprivation," *Proceedings of the Third World Congress in Psychiatry* (1964): 227–31.

13. W. Sargent, *Battle for the Mind* (Garden City, N.Y.: Doubleday, 1957).

14. N. LaBarre, *They Shall Take Up Serpents* (Minneapolis: University Press, 1962).

15. E. Thomas, "The Fire Walk," *Proceedings of the Society for Psychological Research* 42 (1934): 292–309.

16. Peggy Wright, "A Psychobiological Approach to Shamanic Altered States of Consciousness," *ReVision* 16, no. 4 (1994): 164–72.

17. B. Kaplan, *The Inner World of Mental Illness* (New York: Harper, 1964).

18. A. Ludwig, "The Formal Characteristics of Therapeutic Insight," *American Journal of Psychotherapy* 20 (1966): 305–18.

19. Gary Doore, *Shaman's Path* (Boston: Shambhala Publications, 1988).

20. A. Deikman, "The Missing Center," in N. E. Zinberg, (ed.), *Alternate States of Consciousness* (New York: Macmillan, 1977): 230–41.

21. D. Marks, "Intentionality and Autonomy of Verbal Imagery in Altered States of Consciousness," *Behavioral and Brain Science* 9, no. 3 (1986): 529–30.

22. Ibid., p. 529.

23. Nathan Field, "The Therapeutic Function of Altered States," *Journal of Analytic Psychology* 37 (1992): 211–34.

24. A. Mauromatis, "On Shared States of Conscious and Objective Imagery," *Journal of Mental Imagery* 11, no. 2 (1987): 125–30.

25. M. A. Cooperstein, "The Myths of Healing: A Summary of Research into Transpersonal Healing Experiences," *The Journal of the American Society for Psychical Research* 86 (1992): 99–133.

26. Herbert Benson, *The Relaxation Response* (New York: Morrow, 1975).

27. G. Frank Lawlis, David Selby, Glenn Hinnant, and Edward McCoy, "Reduc-

tion of Postoperative Pain Parameters by Presurgical Relaxation Instructions for Spinal Pain Patients," *Spine* 10 (1985): 163–71.

Chapter 6: Imagery

1. A. O. Ransford, D. Cairnes, and V. Mooney, "The Pain Drawing as an Aid to the Psychological Evaluation of Patients with Low Back Pain," *Spine* 2, no. 2, (1976): 127–35.
2. Jeanne Achterberg and G. Frank Lawlis, *Imagery and Disease* (Champaign, Ill.: IPAT, 1984).
3. J. Achterberg, L. Kenner, and G. F. Lawlis, "Severe Burn Injury: A Comparison of Relaxation, Imagery and Biofeedback for Pain Management," *Journal of Mental Imagery* 12, no. 1 (1988): 33–38.
4. D. S. Jacknow, J. M. Tschann, M. P. Link, and W. T. Boyce, "Hypnosis on the Prevention of Chemotherapy-Related Nausea and Vomiting in Children," *Journal of Developmental and Behavioral Pediatrics* 15, no. 4 (1994): 258–64.
5. D. M. Eisenberg, R. C. Kessler, C. Foster, F. E. Norlack, D. R. Calkins, and T. L. Delbanco, "Unconventional Medicine in the United States," *The New England Journal of Medicine* 328, no. 4 (1993): 246–52.
6. Jeanne Achterberg, G. Frank Lawlis, O. Carl Simonton, and Stephanie Simonton, "Psychological Factors and Blood Chemistries as Disease Predictors for Cancer Patients," *Multivariate Clinical Experimental Research* 3, no 3 (1977): 107–22.
7. Jeanne Achterberg, *Imagery in Healing* (Boston: Shambhala Publications, 1985).
8. George Gates, William Ryan, J. C. Cooper, G. Frank Lawlis, Evie Cantu, Toni Hayashi, Edmund Lauder, Richard Welch, and Erwin Hearne, "Current Status of Laryngectomee Rehabilitation I, II, III, IV," *American Journal of Otolaryngology* 3, no. 1 (1982): 1–14, 91–103.
9. John Schneider's research reported in J. Achterberg and G. F. Lawlis, *Imagery and Disease* (Champaign, Ill.: IPAT, 1984), 144–54.
10. Mark Rider, Jeanne Achterberg, G. Frank Lawlis, A. Goven, R. Toledo, and J. R. Butler, "Effects of Immune Systems on Secretory IgA," *Biofeedback and Self-Regulation* 15, no. 4 (1990): 317–32.
11. Mark Rider and Jeanne Achterberg, "The Effect of Music-Mediated Imagery on Neutrophils and Lymphocytes," *Biofeedback and Self-Regulation* 14, no. 3 (1989): 247–57.
12. Steven Gray and G. Frank Lawlis, "A Case Study of Pruritic Eczema Treated by Relaxation and Imagery," *Psychological Reports* 51, no. 3 (1982): 23–28.
13. Howard Hughes, Barry Brown, and G. Frank Lawlis, "Biofeedback-Assisted Relaxation and Imagery for Acne Vulgaris," *Journal of Psychosomatic Research* 27, no. 4 (1983): 16–23.

14. Cheryl Lindberg and G. Frank Lawlis, "The Effectiveness of Imagery as a Childbirth Preparatory Technique," *Journal of Mental Imagery* 12, no. 1 (1988): 31–36.

15. Summarized in J. Achterberg and G. F. Lawlis, *Imagery and Disease* (Champaign, Ill.: IPAT, 1984), pp. 201–35.

16. B. Gruber, N. Hall, S. Hersh, and T. Dubois, "Immune System and Psychological Changes in Metastatic Cancer Patients Using Relaxation and Guided Imagery," *Scandinavian Journal of Behavior Therapy* 17 (1988): 25–46.

17. Jeanne Achterberg, Phillip McGraw, and G. Frank Lawlis, "Rheumatoid Arthritis: A Study of Relaxation and Temperature Biofeedback Training," *Biofeedback and Self-Regulation* 6, no. 2 (1981): 207–23.

18. A. Cott, W. Parkison, W. Fabich, M. Bedard, and R. Marlin, "Long-Term Efficacy of Combined Relaxation and Biofeedback Treatment for Chronic Headache," *Pain* 51, no. 1 (1992): 49–56.

19. J. Achterberg, L. Kenner, and G. F. Lawlis, "Severe Burn Injury: A Comparison of Relaxation, Imagery, and Biofeedback for Pain Management," *Journal of Mental Imagery* 12, no. 1 (1988): 33–38.

20. Jeanne Achterberg, "Imagery and Health," presentation at the Master Teacher Series, Philadelphia: Creative Energies Options, 1993.

21. R. Penrose, *Shadows of the Mind* (New York: Oxford University Press, 1994).

22. J. Achterberg, "Healing Images and Symbols in Nonordinary States of Consciousness," *ReVision* 16, no. 4 (1994): 148–56.

23. A. Arrien, *The Signs of Life* (Sonoma, Calif.: Arcus, 1991).

24. G. Frank Lawlis, *The Cure* (San Jose, Calif.: Resource Publications, 1995).

Chapter 7: Co-consciousness Transformation

1. B. O'Reagan and C. Hirshberg, *Spontaneous Remissions* (Sausalito, Calif.: Institute of Noetic Sciences, 1993).

2. Pierre Janet, *L'Automatisme psychologique* (Paris: Felix Alcan, 1889). M. H. Erickson and E. M. Erickson, "Concerning the Nature and Character of Posthypnotic Behavior," *Journal of General Psychology* 24 (1941): 95–133. F. W. Myers, "Multiplex Personality," *Proceedings of the Society of Psychical Research* 4 (1886): 496–514.

3. M. Prince, *Dissociation of a Personality* (New York: Longman, Green, 1906).

4. J. O. Beahrs, *Unity and Multiplicity* (New York: Brunner/Mazel, 1982). J. O. Beahrs, *Limits of Scientific Psychiatry: The Role of Uncertainty in Mental Health* (New York: Brunner/Mazel, 1986).

5. P. MacLean, *A Triune Concept of the Brain and Behavior* (Toronto: University of Toronto Press, 1973).

6. J. Levy, "Interhemispheric Collaboration: Single-Mindedness in the Asym-

metrical Brain," in C. Best (ed.), *Hemispheric Functions and Collaboration in the Child* (New York: Academic Press, 1985).

7. L. Tinnin, "Obligatory Resistance to Insight," *American Journal of Art Therapy* 28 (1990): 68–70.

8. L. Tinnin, "The Anatomy of the Ego," *Psychiatry* 52 (1989): 404–09.

9. M. Gazzaniga and B. Volpe, "Split-Brain Studies: Implications for Psychiatry," in S. Arieti (ed.), *American Handbook of Psychiatry*, 2nd ed., vol. 7 (New York: Basic Books, 1981).

10. C. G. Jung, *Collected Works*, vol. 18, trans. H. G. Baynes (Princeton, N.J.: Princeton University Press, 1976).

11. H. F. Ellenberger, *The Discovery of the Unconscious: The History and Evolution of Dynamic Psychiatry* (New York: Basic Books, 1970).

12. E. A. Bennet, ed., *What Jung Really Said*, 2nd ed. (New York: Schocken Books, 1983).

13. F. Humbert, *C. G. Jung* (Wilmette, Ill.; Chiron, 1988). B. S. Sullivan, *Psychotherapy Grounded in the Feminine Principle* (Wilmette, Ill.: Chiron, 1989).

14. E. Berne, *Games People Play* (New York: Grove Press, 1964).

15. R. Moore and D. Gillette, *King, Warrior, Magician, and Lover: Rediscovering the Archetypes of the Masculine* (New York: HarperCollins, 1990).

16. H. Storm, *Seven Arrows* (New York: Ballantine Books, 1972).

17. E. Taylor, *William James on Exceptional Mental States: The 1986 Lowell Lectures* (New York: Scribners, 1982).

18. F. W. Putnam, "The Switch Process in Multiple Personality Disorder and Other State-Change Disorders," *Dissociation* 1, no. 1 (1989): 12–16.

19. R. Allison, "A Guide to Parents: How to Raise Your Daughter to Have Multiple Personalities," *Journal of the Family Therapy Insitute of Marin* (Summer 1974): 83–88.

20. E. R. Hilgard, *Divided Consciousness: Multiple Controls in Human Thought and Action* (New York: Wiley, 1977).

21. B. Brown, *Defining the Inner Bag Lady: An Aspect of the Feminine as Experienced by Contemporary Women*, Ph.D. dissertation, Institute of Transpersonal Psychology, Palo Alto, Calif., 1993.

22. M. Murphy and R. White, *The Psychic Side of Sports* (Reading, Mass.: Addison-Wesley, 1978): p. 10.

23. Ibid., p. 29.

24. Ibid., p. 31.

Chapter 8: Death and Transition

1. Stephen Levine, *Who Dies?* (Garden City, N.Y.: Anchor Press/Doubleday, 1982): p. 24.

2. Stephen Levine, *Healing into Life and Death* (New York: Anchor, 1989).

3. Raymond A. Moody, *Life after Life: The Investigation of a Phenomenon—Survival of Bodily Death* (St. Simons Island Geeyo: Mockingbird Books, 1975).
4. Kenneth Ring, *Life at Death: A Scientific Investigation of the Near-Death Experience* (New York: Quill, 1982).
5. August Reader, "The Internal Mystery Plays: The Role and Physiology of the Visual System in Contemplative Practices," *Alternative Therapies* 1, no. 4 (1995): 54–63.
6. J. Schneider, *Stress, Loss and Grief* (Baltimore: University Park Press, 1984).

Chapter 9: Humor and Transformation.

1. Norman Cousins, *Anatomy of an Illness* (New York: Norton, 1979).
2. J. J. Askenasy, "The Functions and Dysfunctions of Laughter," *Journal of General Psychology*, 114, no. 4 (1989): 317–34.
3. Charles Darwin, *Expressions of the Emotions in Man and Animal* (New York: Appleton & Co., 1890).
4. Sigmund Freud, *Jokes and Their Relation to the Unconscious* (New York: Norton, 1960).
5. Gordon W. Allport, *Patterns and Growth in Personality* (New York: Holt, Rinehart & Winston, 1961).
6. Abraham Maslow, Toward a Psychology of Being (New York: Van Nostrand, 1968).
7. Carl Rogers, *On Becoming a Person* (Boston: Houghton Miffin, 1961).
8. Michael Harner, *The Way of the Shaman* (San Francisco: Harper and Row, 1980).
9. H. L. Labrentz, "The Effects of Humor on the Initial Client-Counselor Relationship," Ph.D dissertation, University of Southern Mississippi, *Dissertation Abstracts International* 34 (1974): 3875.
10. A. T. Huber, "The Effect of Humor on Client Discomfort in the Counseling Interview," Ph.D. dissertation, Lehigh University, *Dissertation Abstracts International* 35 (1974): 1980.
11. G. Galon, E. Rosenhein, and J. Jaffe, "Humour in Psychotherapy," *British Journal of Psychotherapy* 4 (1988): 393–400.
12. S. Svebak, "The Effect of Mirthfulness upon Amount of Discordant Right-Left Occipital EEG Alpha," *Motivation and Emotion* 6, no. 2 (1982): 133–46.
13. P. Long, "Laugh and Be Well?" *Psychology Today* (October 1987): 28–29.
14. W. F. Fry, "The Respiratory Components of Mirthful Laughter," *Journal of Biological Psychology* 19, no. 2 (1977): 39–50.
15. D. C. McClelland and C. Kirshait, cited in Daniel Goleman, "The Chicken Soup Effect," *Psychology Today* (October 1982): 80–82.
16. A. J. Chapman and H. C. Foot, *Humor and Laughter: Theory, Research and Applications* (Chichester, England: Wiley, 1976).

17. R. H. Blythe, quoted in Richard Lewis, "Infant Joy," *Parabola* 12, no. 4 (1987): 47.
18. David Goodman (ed.), *Be as You Are: The Teaching of Sri Ramana Maharshi* (London: Routledge & Kegan Paul, 1985).
19. Blythe, in Lewis, "Infant Joy," p. 44.

Chapter 10: Pain as a Doorway to Healing

1. D. D. Kosambi, "Living Prehistory in India," *Scientific American* 216 (1967): 105.
2. C. Wissler, "The Sun Dance of the Blackfoot Indians," *American Museum of Natural History Anthropology Papers* 16 (1921): 437–44.
3. A. L. Kroeber, *Anthropology* (New York: Harcourt, 1948).
4. J. D. Hardy, H. G. Wolff, and H. Goodell, *Pain Sensations and Reactions* (New York: Williams and Wilkins, 1952).
5. R. A. Sternbach and B. Tursky, "Ethnic Differences among Housewives in Psychophysical and Skin Potential Responses to Electric Shock," *Psychophysiology* 1 (1965): 12–14.
6. H. K. Beecher, *Measurement of Subjective Responses* (Oxford: Oxford University Press, 1959).
7. G. Frank Lawlis, Jeanne Achterberg, Linda Kenner, and Kris Kopetz, "Ethnic and Sex Differences in Responses to Pain," *Spine* 9 (1984): 751–54.
8. J. M. Murry, "Ethnicity and Cognitive Complexity of Chronic Pain Patients," Ph.D. dissertation, University of North Texas, Denton, 1990.
9. C. Sargent, "Between Death and Shame: Dimensions of Pain in Bariba Culture," *Social Science and Medicine* 19 (1984): 23–45.
10. A. O. Ransford, D. Cairns, and V. Mooney, "The Pain Drawing as an Aid to the Psychological Evaluation of Patients with Low Back Pain," *Spine* 2 (1976): 127–35.
11. Jeanne Achterberg and G. Frank Lawlis, *Imagery and Disease* (Champaign, Ill.: Institute of Personality and Ability Testing, 1984).
12. Jeanne Achterberg and G. Frank Lawlis, *Health Attribution Test* (Champaign, Ill.: Institute of Personality and Ability Testing, 1989).
13. G. Frank Lawlis, David Selby, Glen Hinnant, and C. Edward McCoy, "Reduction of Postoperative Pain Parameters by Presurgical Relaxation Instructions for Spinal Pain Patients," *Spine* 10 (1985): 163–71.
14. Viktor Frankl, *The Doctor and the Soul* (New York: Knopf, 1960).

INDEX

Universality
  collective unconscious and, 125
  connectedness with, 8
  disease source and, 61
  ritual awareness of, 28
  ritual healing power and, 23
  See also Community; Transpersonal
    moment

Vasiliev, Leonid, 48
Visual imagery, 107
"Voodoo" negative imaging, 53–54, 58,
  62–63

Way of the Shaman, The (Harner), 179
Who Dies? (Levine), 164
"Wounded healer" concept, 201–202

CPSIA information can be obtained at www.ICGtesting.com
Printed in the USA
LVOW10s1838070815

449270LV00002B/377/P